Download the Gunner Goggles App Now!

Go to the App Store from your iPhone or iPad and search for **Gunner Goggles**

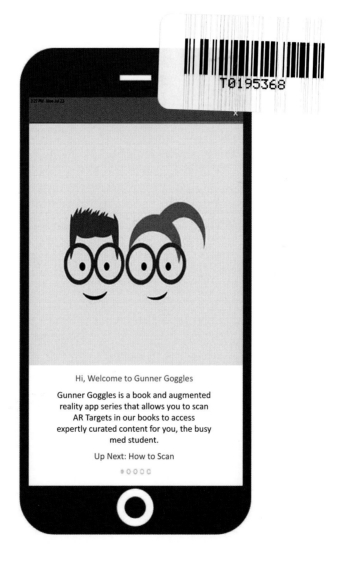

Hi, Welcome to Gunner Goggles

Gunner Goggles is a book and augmented reality app series that allows you to scan AR Targets in our books to access expertly curated content for you, the busy med student.

Up Next: How to Scan

Each Gunner Goggles specialty has its own app; you can purchase other titles at:
ElsevierHealth.com/GunnerGoggles

GUNNER GOGGLES

Obstetrics and Gynecology

HONORS SHELF REVIEW

EDITORS:

Hao-Hua Wu, MD
Resident, Department of
Orthopaedic Surgery
University of California–San Francisco
San Francisco, California

Leo Wang, MS, PhD
Perelman School of Medicine
University of Pennsylvania
Philadelphia, Pennsylvania

Rebecca W. Gao, MS
Stanford University School of Medicine
Stanford, California

FACULTY EDITORS:

Holly W. Cummings, MD, MPH
Assistant Professor of Clinical
Obstetrics and Gynecology
Perelman School of Medicine
University of Pennsylvania
Philadelphia, Pennsylvania

Cynthia DeTata, MD
Clinical Assistant Professor of
Obstetrics and Gynecology
Maternal Fetal Medicine
Stanford Medicine
Stanford, California

DaCarla Albright, MD
Associate Professor of Clinical
Obstetrics and Gynecology
Perelman School of Medicine
University of Pennsylvania
Philadelphia, Pennsylvania

Pam Levin, MD
Assistant Professor of Clinical
Obstetrics and Gynecology
Perelman School of Medicine
University of Pennsylvania
Philadelphia, Pennsylvania

Wanda Ronner, MD
Professor of Clinical Obstetrics and
Gynecology
Perelman School of Medicine
University of Pennsylvania
Philadelphia, Pennsylvania

ELSEVIER

ELSEVIER

1600 John F. Kennedy Blvd.
Ste 1800
Philadelphia, PA 19103-2899

GUNNER GOGGLES OBSTETRICS AND GYNECOLOGY,
HONORS SHELF REVIEW

ISBN: 978-0-323-51037-0

Library of Congress Cataloging-in-Publication Data
Names: Wu, Hao-Hua editor. | Wang, Leo, editor. | Albright, DaCarla, editor.
Title: Gunner goggles obstetrics and gynecology : honors shelf review /
  editors, Hao-Hua Wu, Leo Wang ; faculty editors, DaCarla Albright [and
  four others].
Description: Philadelphia, PA : Elsevier, [2019] | Includes bibliographical
  references.
Identifiers: LCCN 2017051682 | ISBN 9780323510370 (pbk. : alk. paper)
Subjects: | MESH: Obstetrics | Gynecology | Test Taking Skills | Study Guide
Classification: LCC RG101 | NLM WQ 18.2 | DDC 618.1--dc23 LC record
  available at https://lccn.loc.gov/2017051682

Executive Content Strategist: Jim Merritt
Senior Content Development Specialist: Dee Simpson
Publishing Services Manager: Patricia Tannian
Senior Project Manager: Cindy Thoms
Senior Book Designer: Maggie Reid

Printed in China

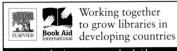

Working together
to grow libraries in
developing countries

www.elsevier.com • www.bookaid.org

Last digit is the print number: 9 8 7 6 5 4 3 2 1

Gunner Goggles Honors Shelf Review Series:

Gunner Goggles Family Medicine	978-0-323-51034-9
Gunner Goggles Medicine	978-0-323-51035-6
Gunner Goggles Neurology	978-0-323-51036-3
Gunner Goggles Obstetrics and Gynecology	978-0-323-51037-0
Gunner Goggles Pediatrics	978-0-323-51038-7
Gunner Goggles Psychiatry	978-0-323-51039-4
Gunner Goggles Surgery	978-0-323-51040-0

Contributors

Gerald Michael Baer, MD
Resident Physician
Department of Neurology
University of Pennsylvania
Philadelphia, Pennsylvania
Systemic Disorders Affecting Pregnancy, Labor and Delivery, and the Puerperium

Esther Baranov, MD
Resident Physician
Department of Pathology
Brigham & Women's Hospital
Boston, Massachusetts
Neoplasms of the Ovary, Uterus, Cervix, Vagina, and Vulva

Sierra Centkowski, MD
Resident Physician
Department of Dermatology
Stanford University School of Medicine
Palo Alto, California
Systemic Disorders Affecting Pregnancy, Labor and Delivery, and the Puerperium

Drake Lebrun, MD, MPH
Resident Physician
Department of Orthopaedic Surgery
Hospital for Special Surgery
New York, New York
Breast Pathologies

Kumar Nadhan
Temple University School of Medicine
Philadelphia, Pennsylvania
Fertility, Infertility, and Birth Control
Menopause
Sexual Dysfunction
Congenital Disorders
Adverse Effects of Drugs on the Female Reproductive System
Adverse Effects of Drugs on Pregnancy, Childbirth, and the Puerperium

Angela Ester Ugorets, MD
Resident Physician
Emergency Medicine
Cooper University
Camden, New Jersey
Infections of the Female Reproductive System

Acknowledgments

"If I have seen further than others, it is by standing upon the shoulders of giants."

– Isaac Newton

We would like to thank the many exceptional innovators who helped transform our vision of *Gunner Goggles Obstetrics and Gynecology* into reality.

To our editorial team at Elsevier, thank you for your unrelenting support throughout the publication process. Jim Merritt believed in *Gunner Goggles* from day one and used his experience as an executive content strategist to point us in the right direction with respect to book proposal, product pitch, and manuscript development. Dee Simpson expertly guided us through manuscript submission and revision, no easy feat with two first-time authors. Maggie Reid collaborated with us closely to create the layout design and color schemes. Cindy Thoms and the copy editing team made sure our written content adhered to a high professional standard.

To the editors, authors, and student reviewers of *Gunner Goggles Obstetrics and Gynecology*, thank you for your scholarship and unwavering enthusiasm. Our outstanding faculty editors—Dr. Holly Cummings, Dr. Cynthia DeTata, Dr. DaCarla Albright, Dr. Wanda Ronner, Dr. Pamela Levin—took time out of their busy schedules to meticulously edit each chapter provide numerous invaluable insights on how to improve quality and accuracy. A number of outstanding residents and medical students contributed to the content of this textbook and provided us feedback on high-yield topics for the NBME Obstetrics and Gynecology Subject Exam, notably Dr. Michael Baer, Dr. Esther Baranov, Dr. Sierra Centkowski, Dr. Drake Lebrun, Dr. Kumar Nadhan, and Dr. Angela Ugorets.

To our augmented reality (AR) team, thank you for your creativity and dedication during the development of the *Gunner Goggles* AR application. Nadir Bilici, Brian Mayo, Vlad Obsekov, Clare Teng, and Yinka Orafidiya helped us develop and test the initial *Gunner Goggles* AR prototype. Tammy Bui designed the *Gunner Goggles* logo and AR app icon.

We would also like to thank the Wharton Innovation Fund for awarding us seed money to help pursue development of *Gunner Goggles* AR.

You all continue to inspire us, and we are incredibly grateful and deeply appreciative for your support.

– Hao-Hua, Leo, and Rebecca

Contents

Introduction

Hao-Hua Wu and Leo Wang

I. Gunner's Guide to a Better Test Score

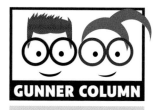

GUNNER COLUMN

Curious why certain classmates perform well on every exam? Frustrated by how few of these "Gunner" peers share study secrets?

At *Gunner Goggles*, our goal is to reveal and demystify. By integrating *augmented reality* into this review book, we **reveal** how the best students approach topics, conceptualize complex disease, and allocate study time efficiently. By organizing each topic according to the National Board of Medical Examiners (NBME) format, we **demystify** exam content and the types of questions you can expect on test day.

Of the tests medical students strive to conquer, shelf exams boast the highest ratio of importance to study resource quality. For instance, performance on shelf exams typically informs final clerkship grades, which are the most important criteria on the medical school transcript for residency application. Yet there is no single authoritative study resource for the shelf across all disciplines. Most importantly, no current book specifically targets shelf exam prep. Thus students must rely on miscellaneous resources and anecdotal advice to get the job done.

In light of this void in authoritative test prep, we have created the *Gunner Goggles* series to provide you with the most effective shelf exam testing resource. *GG* stands out for three important reasons:

First, readers have the opportunity to enhance their understanding of important shelf topics by utilizing the **augmented reality (AR)** features on each page. With an iPhone or iPad, users can download the *Gunner Goggles* AR iOS app and use it to turn book figures into three-dimensional (3D) images, access high-yield videos and view pertinent digital media. More on how AR technology works can be found on page 2.

Second, *Gunner Goggles* provides a plethora of tips on how to manage time efficiently in studying for the shelf. Mnemonics and strategies for how to approach difficult concepts can be found in the blue Gunner Column on each page. We also tell you how to *think* about these concepts so that obstetrics/gynecology (OB/Gyn) never feels like a laundry list of items you simply have to memorize.

Third, this review book is written and organized optimally for shelf exam test prep. Each chapter is organized according to the NBME Clinical Science Subject Examination and USMLE Course Content outlines. In addition, a concise summary of how topics are tested prefaces each chapter.

As experts on the shelf exam, we understand how difficult it is to carve out time to study while juggling clinical responsibilities during your clerkship rotation. We also know that each student's learning curve is different based on timing of the rotation (first block vs. last block), year in medical school (MS3 vs. MD/PhD returning after graduate school), and future career interests (e.g., an aspiring orthopedic surgeon learning about obstetrics and gynecology). However, we believe that any student can perform well on the shelf with the right strategy and study resources.

We created this book anticipating the needs of all types of students, and hope that *Gunner Goggles* will be the most comprehensive, authoritative shelf exam review book that you ever use. We are confident that *Gunner Goggles* will enable you to achieve your test performance goals and stick it to your "Gunner" classmates, whose advice, or lack thereof, you won't be needing after all.

II. Augmented Reality: A New Paradigm for Shelf Exam Test Prep

Think of AR as your best friend.

To use it, download the free *Gunner Goggles Obstetrics and Gynecology* application on your iPad or iPhone and create your own optional profile. Now, with the application open, point your smart mobile camera at this page.

Notice how on your camera, there are now links you can click on, 3D figures you can rotate, and a video you can watch. You have just unlocked the AR features for this page!

Take a moment to play around with these AR features on your smart mobile device. The way it works is this: anytime you see the *Gunner Goggles* icon **gg** in the blue Gunner Column at the right, there is an AR feature accompanying the text. You have the opportunity to interact with that.

Still not convinced? Here are three reasons why AR is your ideal study companion.

Presentation

AR breaks the boundaries of how information can be presented in a textbook.

gg AR
Introduction Video

gg AR
Contact

Traditionally, if you wanted to learn about a disease in a review book, you would be expected to read and memorize a block of text similar to the following:

Huntington's disease (HD) is a GABAergic neurodegenerative disorder that is caused by an autosomal dominant mutation leading to CAG repeats on chromosome 4. Patients typically present in the fourth and fifth decade of life with chorea, memory loss, caudate atrophy on neuroimaging, and motor impairment, depending on the variant. Although there is no cure for Huntington's, the movement disorders associated with the disease, such as chorea, can be treated with drugs like tetrabenazine and reserpine to decrease dopamine release.

Having read (or most likely glazed) through that paragraph, do you feel comfortable enough to answer questions about the genetics, presentation, and treatment of Huntington disease right now? A week from now? Three weeks from now when you have to take your shelf exam?

Here's where AR comes in. Use your *Gunner Goggles* app to check out how we're able to present Huntington disease in different, memorable ways.

For visual learners, here's a video of an effective Huntington disease mnemonic →

If you are an audio learner, here's a link to key points about Huntington disease for the shelf →

Forgot your neuroanatomy? Here's where the caudate is →

What's the difference between chorea, athetosis, and ballismus again? Chorea looks like this →

Now write a one-line description of Huntington disease in your own words in the margins of this page for future reference. It's much easier with AR right? Like we said, your best friend.

9g AR

Huntington Disease

9g AR

Huntington's Podcast

9g AR

The caudate nucleus is part of the basal ganglia

9g AR

Chorea patient example

Evaluation

The GG Obstetrics and Gynecology app has the potential to exponentially enhance how you can evaluate your own understanding of the material. Although not available with the first edition, we are in the process of developing a personalized question bank as well as a flashcards feature. Our vision is to allow you to scan a topic on the page for immediate access to relevant practice questions and flashcards. In future versions, you will also be able to create your own flashcard deck and track your mastery.

In addition the GG app can keep track of the AR Targets scanned and the Learning links viewed. These links are saved to a Link Library which you can view at any time. You can also like or dislike a Learning Link with an opportunity to provide us feedback for better resources available.

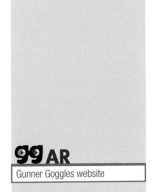

As development of the GG Obstetrics and Gynecology app is an ongoing process, we encourage and welcome your feedback. If you like the idea of having a personalized question bank and flashcard feature or have an idea for how we can improve the GG app to better serve your studying needs, please provide us feedback through an in-app message. You can also email us at GunnerGoggles@gmail.com.

Community Engagement

Studying for the shelf can be isolating. Our vision is to develop a feature in the GG Obstetrics and Gynecology that would allow you to connect with chapter authors and fellow readers. We are in the process of developing a medium in which shelf-related inquiries can be discussed among authors and readers through an optional short message system (SMS) feature.

Given that the community engagement feature is in development and unavailable for the first edition, we welcome your input on how we can connect you with the people who will enable your test day success.

To provide feedback, please scan the page and vote. You can also email us GunnerGoggles@gmail.com for any comments or suggestions.

Augmented Reality Frequently Asked Questions

"Since augmented reality is integrated into *Gunner Goggles OB/Gyn*, does this mean I have to pull out my iPad or iPhone for every page of the book?"

No, only if you need it. Some may use AR more than others, depending on background and level of comfort with the material. For instance, you may already have a solid understanding of polycystic ovarian syndrome (PCOS) and need to read the text only as a refresher. On the other hand, if you are less comfortable with PCOS, the digital media featured with AR are there just in case.

"Can't I just look up everything I don't know on my own? Why do I have to use the *Gunner Goggles* app?"

You can absolutely look things up on your own. But that takes time. And sometimes, you can't find the best reference or mnemonic. Our team of experts has already gone through the trouble of identifying potential sources of confusion for you and found the perfect resources. In the *Gunner Goggles* app, we have compiled the slickest and most concise resources one can use to better understand a topic. Videos, audio files, and images are first vetted by subject experts for accuracy of content. They are then evaluated by students like you for utility of content to enhance test performance. Only resources with the most Gunner votes are embedded into each page.

"What if a link doesn't work or I want something on the page to change?"

Please tell us! Another advantage of AR is that we can immediately receive and implement your feedback. Just use the *Gunner Goggles* app to text us your concerns and our tech support team will respond ASAP!

III. Study Smart: Mnemonics and Gunner Study Tips

Even with incredible AR features at your disposal, you won't be able to optimize exam performance unless you know how to study. Below are the four most important things one can do to study for the OB/Gyn shelf under the time restraints imposed by clerkships.

Understand the Organizing Principle

The easiest way to save time and perform well on the shelf is to understand how a specific disease or concept fits into the big picture. For instance, knowing the buzz words, diagnostic steps, and treatment plan for endometriosis will likely lead to only one correct answer on the test. However, understanding how endometriosis fits into the spectrum of disorders that cause chronic pelvic pain (e.g., adenomyosis, fibroids, etc.) can help you to quickly evaluate a complaint of pelvic discomfort.

Create Effective Mnemonics

If you have a photographic memory, skip this section. For the rest of us mere mortals, the organizing principles (OPs) of what constitutes a Gunner mnemonic are outlined below.

Mnemonics are important when:
a. You have to learn a lot of material.
b. You want to teach something to your colleagues during morning rounds. Attendings and residents are always impressed when they can learn something from a medical student.
c. You want to remember something 15 years from now when you are working the 30th hour of a busy call day.

OPs for mnemonics are as follows:

1. Use the spelling of a name to your benefit **(Spell)**.
   Example:
   a. "8urk14tt" lymphoma (Burkitt lymphoma), lep"thin" (leptin), "supraoptiuretic" nuclei (supraoptic nuclei that produce antidiuretic hormone)
   b. Tenofovir is the only NRTI nucleoTide
   c. We"C"ener granulomatosis (GPA) for C-ANCA and Cyclophosphamide tx
2. Create an acronym that contains distinguishing syllables or letters of names **(Distinguish)**.
   Example:
   a. Chronic Alcoholics Steal PhenPhen and Nevar Rifuse Grisee Carbs (<u>Chronic alcohol</u> abuse + St. John's wort + phenytoin + phenobarb + nevaripine + rifampin + griseofulvin + carbamazepine):
      • Reinforce a mnemonic by spelling the name of the item to be memorized accordingly.
      • For example, "Refus"ampin, "Never"apine, "Greasy"ofulvin, "Carb"amazepine, etc.
      • This ties mnemonic OP 1 with mnemonic OP 2.
3. Drawings help **(Draw)**.
   Example: Trisomy 13 looks like polydactyly + cleft lip when the number 13 is rotated 90 degrees clockwise (the horizontal 1 is the extra digit, and the cleft of the horizontal 3 is the cleft lip).
4. Counting the letters of a word **(Count)**.
   Example: Patau syndrome = 13 letters = Trisomy 13
5. Arrange acronym in alphabetical order **(Arrange)**.
   Example: ABCDEF for diphtheria (ADP ribosylation, beta prophage, C Diphtheria, elongation factor 2).

Examples of instructors who practice this concept well are Dr. John Barone of Kaplan and Dr. Husain Sattar of Pathoma.

On the flip side, here are examples of poor mnemonics (although you may remember them now, given that they are highlighted in this text):

a. Blind as a bat, mad as a hatter, red as a beet, hot as Hades, dry as a bone, the bowel and bladder lose their tone, and the heart runs alone = poor mnemonic for anticholinergic syndrome:
   • This mnemonic forces you to memorize extra and extraneous things (like bat, beet, hare, and desert) which have nothing to do with anticholinergic syndrome.
b. WWHHHHIMP (withdrawal + Wernicke + hypertensive crisis + hypoxia + hypoglycemia + hypoperfusion +

99 AR
Trisomy 13

intracranial bleed + meningitis/encephalopathy + poisoning) = poor mnemonic for causes of delirium:

- Wait, how many H's does this mnemonic have again?

A good rule of thumb: If you can still remember a mnemonic in a high-pressure situation (attending pimps you) or after a 7-day period, then you have a winner.

Ultimately, the best mnemonics are the ones you invent and apply repeatedly. So use these mnemonic principles to give yourself a solid head start.

Devise a Study Schedule and Stick to It

The third most important piece of advice for the shelf is to create a study schedule at the beginning of the rotation and follow it. Rotations such as OB/Gyn are particularly draining. Often you may find yourself coming home after a 12-hour shift on Gyn/Onc and not wanting to study, especially when pre-rounds are the next day at 5 a.m. However, if you are mentally committed to following a schedule, you will find creative ways to get the studying done. For example, some students wake up an hour early to read before prerounds. Others fit study material into their white coats and read during downtime. OB/Gyn is unique because you are almost guaranteed to have downtime in between cases. Take that opportunity to peruse notes and do shelf practice questions on your cell phone.

Distinguish Rotation Knowledge from Shelf Knowledge

Many of the things you learn on rotation do not apply to the shelf exam and vice versa. For example, you may be able to impress your OB/Gyn attending by committing the prevalence of endometrial cancer in the United States to memory. However, with only 150 minutes to answer 100 lengthy questions on the shelf, details like that have no utility. Be able to compartmentalize and know exactly what is needed for your OB/Gyn rotation and what is expected on the shelf to save yourself precious study time.

IV. Intro to the National Board of Medical Examiners Clinical Science Obstetrics/Gynecology Subject Exam

The Clinical Science OB/Gyn NBME Shelf Exam is a 110-question computerized exam administered over a recommended course of 2 hours and 45 minutes, typically at

99 AR

NBME Shelf Exam Website

the conclusion of your OB/Gyn clerkship rotation. The test questions come from either retired step 2 CK questions or are written by a committee of faculty across the country. Thus it is important to master shelf exam–style questions to set yourself up nicely for step 2 CK.

Unlike step 1, shelf exam questions focus almost exclusively on disease processes rather than normal processes. That being said, the most high-yield normal processes to know for the OB/Gyn shelf are the menstrual cycle, fetal gestation, and labor and delivery.

According to the NBME, the exams are curved to a mean of 70 with a standard deviation of 8. The curve does not take into account timing of rotation. For instance, students who take the exam during their first clerkship block will be held to the same statistical standard as students who take the exam during their fourth block. However, the NBME does release "quarterly norm information" to medical schools in order to make clerkship directors aware of the relationship between exam score and rotation timing.

Although different OB/Gyn clerkships have different standards for determining grades, many programs have a cutoff score that must be achieved to qualify for the highest clerkship grade (e.g., honors). If this is the case, confirm the cutoff score with your clerkship director so that you have a reasonable performance goal to shoot for.

Every question on the OB/Gyn shelf will ask you about one of four things: (1) protocol for promoting health maintenance (Prophylaxis [**PPx**]), (2) the mechanism of disease (**MoD**), (3) steps to establishing a diagnosis (**Dx**), and (4) steps of disease management (**Tx/Mgmt**). The frequency with which you can expect these "Physician Tasks" to appear as shelf questions can be found here:

General Principles, Including Normal Age-Related Findings and Care of the Well Patient	1%–5%
Pregnancy, Childbirth, and the Puerperium	40%–45%
Female Reproductive System and Breast	40%–45%
Endocrine System	1%–5%
Other Systems, Including Multisystem Processes and Disorders	5%–10%
Social Sciences	1%–5%

The two main categories, "Pregnancy, Childbirth, and the Puerperium" (a.k.a., Obstetrics) and "Female Reproductive System and Breast" (a.k.a., Gynecology) are further subdivided into the following content:

Pregnancy, Childbirth, and the Puerperium

a. Preconception counseling and care
b. Prenatal risk assessment/prevention
c. Supervision of normal pregnancy
d. Obstetric complications
e. Labor and delivery
f. Puerperium, including complications
g. Newborn (birth to 4 weeks of age)
h. Congenital disorders, neonatal
i. Adverse effects of drugs on pregnancy, childbirth, and the puerperium
j. Systemic disorders affecting pregnancy, labor and delivery, and the puerperium

Female Reproductive System and Breast

a. Normal processes, female function (e.g., ovulation, menstrual cycle, puberty)
b. Breast: infectious, immunologic, and inflammatory disorders
c. Neoplasms of breast
d. Female reproductive: infectious, immunologic, and inflammatory disorders
e. Neoplasms of cervix, ovary, uterus, vagina, and vulva
f. Fertility and infertility
g. Menopause
h. Menstrual and endocrine disorders
i. Sexual dysfunction
j. Traumatic and mechanical disorders
k. Congenital disorders
l. Adverse effects of drugs on the female reproductive system and breast

Currently, the NBME Obstetrics and Gynecology Content Outline breaks down question types into these categories:

- Applying Foundational Science Concepts (8%–12%)
- Diagnosis: Knowledge Pertaining to History, Exam, Diagnostic Studies, and Patient Outcomes (45%–50%)
- Health Maintenance, Pharmacotherapy, Intervention, and Management (33%–42%)

However, devising a study plan from these three categories can be confusing. "Applying Foundational Science Concepts," for instance, is vague and difficult to prepare for. Instead, many students prefer to study according to Physician Tasks provided in older content outlines. Since every subject exam question asks about one of four things— (1) protocol for promoting health maintenance (Prophylaxis

[PPx]), (2) the mechanism of disease (MoD), (3) steps to establishing a diagnosis (Dx), and (4) steps of disease management (Tx/Mgmt)—we recommend studying according to Physician Tasks from the 2016 Content Outline.

Physician Tasks (from 2016 Content Outline)

Promoting Health and Health Maintenance	10%–20%
Understanding Mechanisms of Disease	30%–40%
Establishing a Diagnosis	30%–40%
Applying Principles of Management	10%–20%

In addition, the NBME breaks down questions by Site of Care, including:
- Ambulatory (70%–75%)
- Emergency Department (5%–10%)
- Inpatient (15%–20%)

Our recommendation is to not worry about site of care and focus on studying content related to Physician Tasks.

Each disease is also presented in a "PPx, MoD, Dx, and Tx/Mgmt" format, which represents the four physician tasks the NBME can test you on. Since establishing a diagnosis is weighted especially heavily (15%–20%), a "Buzz Words" category has been added to show you how to quickly identify the disease process from just a few key words. A "Clinical Presentation" section has also been added to describe the disease more thoroughly. However, it is important to note that buzz words are sufficient to correctly identify the corresponding disease on the shelf. The detail provided in the Clinical Presentation section is meant to only augment your understanding, particularly if it is your first pass. However, by the end of studying, the focus should primarily be on buzz words.

Finally, here are five main things to keep in mind while studying for the OB/Gyn shelf:
1. If pressed for time, practice identifying disease processes only through buzz words. For instance, on the shelf exam, a patient with a uterus that has a "snowstorm" appearance on ultrasound will likely have a hydatidiform mole (e.g., gestational trophoblastic disease).
2. "Tx/Mgmt" details of gynecologic disorders are less frequently tested than "Tx/Mgmt" of obstetrics disorders (5%–10% vs. 10%–15%). This is because many of the surgical procedures for treating gynecologic neoplasms are beyond the scope of this exam. Thus focus less on learning fancy surgical techniques and more on the treatment of breast disorders and sexually transmitted infections.

3. Know your medicine! One of the biggest mistakes that people make in studying for the OB/Gyn Shelf is assuming that only OB/Gyn diseases can be tested. However, some of the questions on the OB/Gyn shelf are taken from the Medicine shelf but may have a chief complaint that connotes OB/Gyn pathology (e.g., "lower abdominal pain" could be GI vs. OB/Gyn). Therefore make sure to learn the medical disorders that affect pregnant women (Chapter 19), as medicine concepts show up on multiple shelf exams.

4. Make sure to begin doing questions early (e.g., 10 questions a day starting from day 1). Ideally you should make a second pass at the most high-yield questions before test day.

5. For each question, write a one-line take-home point in an Excel spreadsheet. This makes for quick and easy review in the days leading up to the exam.

If any questions arise while you are studying, use the *Gunner Goggles* app to access the AR features embedded on each page.

Good luck and happy hunting.

—The Gunner Goggles Team

General Principles

Hao-Hua Wu, Leo Wang, Rebecca W. Gao, and Holly W. Cummings

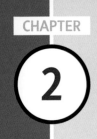

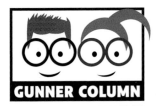

GUNNER COLUMN

Introduction

General principles appear in one to five questions on your Obstetrics/Gynecology (Ob/Gyn) shelf; they focus on normal processes, such as what normal pregnancy looks like. These questions can be tricky because the other 95%–99% of the shelf tests abnormal processes. By the end of this chapter, be sure to know what physiologic changes a woman can experience during normal pregnancy and what types of ethical scenarios you should to be aware of.

This chapter is divided into (1) General Knowledge, (2) Normal Pregnancy, (3) Ethics in Ob/Gyn, and (4) Gunner Practice. Anticipate spending 2–4 hours perusing this chapter for your first pass and make sure to refer to the list of physiologic changes during pregnancy throughout your rotation.

General Knowledge

This section provides an overview of basic terminology you will need to be familiar with to answer Ob/Gyn questions on the shelf. Like psychiatry, Ob/Gyn is so specialized that there is a lot of terminology that you must know in order to apply the concepts effectively.

Note that none of the material covered in this subsection will be directly tested. You will never be asked, for instance, to define the "first trimester" on the shelf. If you are already familiar with Ob/Gyn terminology, skip to the section headed "Normal Pregnancy." Quickly browse this section if you have yet to start your Ob/Gyn rotation or want a quick refresher of foundational definitions.

Gravidity and Parity

Gravidity and parity (abbreviated G and P) are terms that describe obstetric history.

Gravidity is the number of times the patient has been pregnant: G0 = nulligravida (never pregnant), G1 = primigravida (pregnant once), G2 or higher = multigravida (pregnant more than once).

99 AR

High-yield terms from ACOG

Parity is the number of times the patient has carried a baby to a viable gestational age, defined as 20 weeks. P0 = never carried ≥20 weeks, P1 = carried 1 pregnancy ≥20 weeks, P2 = carried 2 pregnancies ≥20 weeks, etc. Twins, triplets, etc., are counted as one pregnancy.

Examples:
- A 23-year-old gravida 2 para 2 woman = 2 pregnancies, 2 pregnancies carried past 20 weeks.
- A 40-year-old G8 P0, woman = 8 pregnancies, 0 pregnancies carried past 20 weeks.

Buzz Words: Gravidity greater than parity (e.g., G3P0 or G2P1) means that the patient has had a previous spontaneous abortion. The number of spontaneous abortions = G − P. So if a patient is G3P1, the number of spontaneous abortions is 2 (i.e., 3 − 1 = 2).

A high number of spontaneous abortions (e.g., G8P0) means that disorders such as antiphospholipid syndrome must be considered.

For the Wards, **term infants, premature infants, abortions, living children (TPAL) and abortions (A)** are sometimes combined with G and P. On notes, you may see something like G1 P 1-0-0-1 (1 pregnancy to term, 0 preterm, 0 abortions, 1 living), or G2P1A1 (e.g., 2 pregnancies, 1 carried past 20 weeks, 1 spontaneous abortion). These are notations that are not seen on the shelf exam, so these are not covered. However, if you understand what this terminology means you will be better able to interpret charts in clinic and to present to your obstetric attendings.

Trimesters

The questions on the shelf exam will never tell you what trimester the mother is in. Instead, you must determine this information through gestational age:
- First trimester: 0–13 weeks:
  - **Most reliable fetal age with transvaginal ultrasound.**
  - Normal processes: spotting/bleeding upon implantation, nausea/vomiting, morning sickness, fatigue, mood swings, breast engorgement and tenderness, fetal heartbeat starting at 6–8 weeks on Doppler fetal monitor, placenta begins to extend into wall of uterus.
- Second trimester: 14–27 weeks:
  - Normal processes: abdominal pain, back pain, gastroesophageal reflux disease (GERD).
- Third trimester: ≥28 weeks:
  - **Least reliable fetal age with transvaginal ultrasound.**

QUICK TIPS
Spontaneous abortion = when fetus becomes nonviable before 20 weeks.

FOR THE WARDS
TPAL, GPA, and other useful terminology for Ob/Gyn rotation

99 AR
ACOG FAQ, what to expect during trimesters of pregnancy

- Normal processes: dyspnea, varicose veins, swelling of hands and feet

Thus, the first part of a question stem on the Ob/Gyn Shelf (e.g., A 23-year-old, gravida 2, para 1, female at 35 weeks' gestation) can tell you a lot about your patient and will indicate whether or not you are dealing with an Ob or a Gyn problem.

Normal Pregnancy

You are guaranteed to have at least a couple of questions about normal pregnancy on the shelf. These questions will come in the form of question stems that pick the most extreme signs and symptoms of pregnancy (i.e., systolic murmur, vaginal spotting or bleeding in the first trimester, increased total T3 and T4, spider angiomata) as the patient's chief complaint to scare you into thinking that this is an abnormal pregnancy. Sometimes, the patient will come in without knowing that she is pregnant. Other times, you will be given the gestational age and asked if the signs/symptoms are appropriate. Do not be fooled. The two easiest ways to distinguish normal from abnormal on the shelf are to determine (1) the effect on everyday function (e.g., complaints with no effect on work/play = normal) and (2) the extent to which the physical exam is abnormal (e.g., enlarged uterus, soft cervix, blue vagina but no other findings/tenderness = normal). See Fig. 2.1 for normal physiologic changes of pregnancy.

Buzz Words: Childbearing age + missed last period + nausea/vomiting + enlarged, engorged breasts + soft enlarged uterus (Hegar sign) + soft "friable" cervix (Goodell sign) + bluish vagina and cervix (Chadwick sign) → normal pregnancy

Clinical Presentation: Ask about the patient's last menstrual period (LMP). If she has menses in a regular cycle (e.g., once every 28 days) and her period is now late, you should always evaluate with a urine pregnancy test.

The main physiologic changes of pregnancy are as follows:
- **Skin**: Because of increases in estrogen and progesterone, spider angiomas and palmar erythema can be found. Owing to increases in melanocyte-stimulating hormone, darkening of the skin (i.e., melasma, dark line in groin/armpit, dark marks on the face, or darkening of the linea nigra on the abdomen) can occur.

FOR THE WARDS

Although fetal development is not tested on the shelf, here's a resource that you can use on your Ob/Gyn rotation:

QUICK TIPS

All patients of childbearing age on the shelf should be evaluated with a urine pregnancy test.

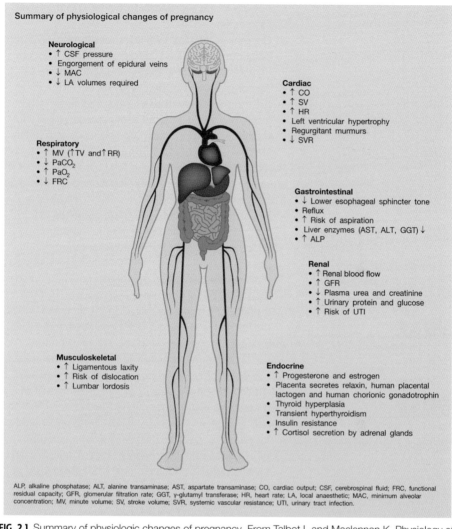

Summary of physiological changes of pregnancy

Neurological
- ↑ CSF pressure
- Engorgement of epidural veins
- ↓ MAC
- ↓ LA volumes required

Cardiac
- ↑ CO
- ↑ SV
- ↑ HR
- Left ventricular hypertrophy
- Regurgitant murmurs
- ↓ SVR

Respiratory
- ↑ MV (↑TV and↑RR)
- ↓ PaCO₂
- ↑ PaO₂
- ↓ FRC

Gastrointestinal
- ↓ Lower esophageal sphincter tone
- Reflux
- ↑ Risk of aspiration
- Liver enzymes (AST, ALT, GGT) ↓
- ↑ ALP

Renal
- ↑ Renal blood flow
- ↑ GFR
- ↓ Plasma urea and creatinine
- ↑ Urinary protein and glucose
- ↑ Risk of UTI

Musculoskeletal
- ↑ Ligamentous laxity
- ↑ Risk of dislocation
- ↑ Lumbar lordosis

Endocrine
- ↑ Progesterone and estrogen
- Placenta secretes relaxin, human placental lactogen and human chorionic gonadotrophin
- Thyroid hyperplasia
- Transient hyperthyroidism
- Insulin resistance
- ↑ Cortisol secretion by adrenal glands

ALP, alkaline phosphatase; ALT, alanine transaminase; AST, aspartate transaminase; CO, cardiac output; CSF, cerebrospinal fluid; FRC, functional residual capacity; GFR, glomerular filtration rate; GGT, γ-glutamyl transferase; HR, heart rate; LA, local anaesthetic; MAC, minimum alveolar concentration; MV, minute volume; SV, stroke volume; SVR, systemic vascular resistance; UTI, urinary tract infection.

FIG. 2.1 Summary of physiologic changes of pregnancy. From Talbot L and Maclennan K. Physiology of pregnancy. *Anaesth Intensive.* 2016;17(7):341-345.

- **Musculoskeletal (MSK):** Patients may suffer from increased lumbar lordosis (the inward curving of the spine) which leads to **lower back pain.**
- **Uterus, cervix, vagina:** On pelvic exam, the three cardinal signs of pregnancy are:
  - Soft enlarged uterus (Hegar sign)
  - Soft friable cervix (Goodell sign)
  - Bluish vagina and cervix (Chadwick sign)
- **Cardiovascular:**
  - An enlarged uterus can compress the inferior vena cava, a phenomenon exacerbated by sleeping in the right decubitus position, leading to less blood

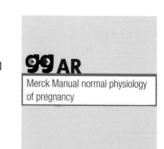

99 AR

Merck Manual normal physiology of pregnancy

flowing to the heart and more edema in the lower extremities.

- Decreased systemic vascular resistance (SVR) from placental circulation → decreased blood pressure (hypotension), commonly in the second trimester.
- To compensate for the energy needs of the fetus, the mother's heart beats harder and faster (e.g., increased stroke volume and increased heart rate = increased cardiac output). This leads to a higher incidence of **systolic murmurs.**
- **Heme:** There is an increase in total blood volume and an **absolute** increase in both plasma and red blood cell (RBC) mass in the mother:
  - Increases in RBC mass and the demands of the fetus create a higher iron requirement, which necessitates iron supplementation during pregnancy.
  - However, patients can be **anemic** (low hemoglobin) on a CBC because the mother's plasma volume increases at a greater rate than the increase in RBC mass. This is known as "dilutional anemia."
- **Pulmonary:** Progesterone increases tidal volume without altering respiratory rate to blow off the extra CO_2 produced by the fetus. On exam, you may see the patient breathing heavily or hear a complaint of dyspnea. This leads to respiratory alkalosis.
- **Renal:**
  - Increased urinary frequency, retention, and risk of pyelonephritis during pregnancy. These are the three urologic conditions most commonly seen on the shelf.
  - In addition, owing to the increased blood volume, glomerular filtration rate (GFR) increases during pregnancy and blood urea nitrogen (BUN) and creatinine (Cr) accordingly decrease. However, these lab values are not frequently tested because *decreased BUN/Cr* are not really buzz words for any other Ob/Gyn condition.
- **Endocrine:**
  - The most high-yield endocrine change is the increase in **human placental lactogen (hPL),** which increases insulin resistance and is a possible cause of gestational diabetes.
  - Elevated total T3, T4, and thyroid-binding globulin circulating in the blood, although free T3 and T4 levels remain the same. Be wary of normal pregnancy questions that try to insinuate thyroid pathology.

gg AR
Physiologic change in pregnancy, Khan Academy

gg AR
Respiratory physiology in pregnancy

- Estrogen, progesterone, and human chorionic gonadotropin (hCG) are also elevated in pregnancy. Beta-hCG increases at a steady rate in the first 10 weeks of pregnancy, but abnormalities either in the rate of increase or the absolute level can be indicative of pathology (e.g., gestational hydatidiform mole or ectopic pregnancy).
- **Gastrointestinal:**
  - The most common GI-related complaints in pregnancy are morning sickness, nausea, and vomiting. Rarely, patients can develop severe nausea and vomiting, known as hyperemesis gravidarum.
  - For the shelf, keep an eye out for abnormal lab values such as an increased alkaline phosphatase level, which is due to placental production and not liver dysfunction; in other words, an increased alkaline phosphatase level is normal in pregnancy.
  - Other GI-related topics that may show up on the question stem are GERD and constipation, the former from relaxation of the lower esophageal sphincter and the latter from compression of the rectum by the enlarged uterus and from muscle relaxation caused by increased progesterone.

This may be a lot of information, but a great mnemonic to use is SMUCH PREGi (pronounced "Smooch Preggi").

Mnemonic: SMUCH PREGi (pronounced Smooch Preggi)

Skin: palmar erythema, spider angiomata, darkening of skin (melasma)

Musculoskletal: hyperlordosis (low back pain)

Uterus: soft, enlarged uterus, spotting/bleeding at 4 weeks due to implantation, cervix soft on exam, bluish vagina

Cardiovascular: increased CO, HR, SV, systolic murmur; decreased BP

Heme: hypercoagulable state, dilutional anemia, normal MCV

Pulmonary: increased tidal volume → increased CO_2 leaving body → respiratory alkalosis, RR stays the same

Renal: increased GFR, increased risk for pyelonephritis (2/2 stasis of urine in ureters from mass effect), increased urinary frequency/urgency

Endocrine: increased estrogen, progesterone, **total T3/T4/thyroid-binding globulin**, hPL and hCG, normal free T3/T4

Gastrointestinal: increased GERD, alkaline phosphatase levels, nausea/vomiting, morning sickness, constipation

Hyperemesis gravidarum Merck Manual

MNEMONIC

SMUCH PREGi
Skin
Musculoskeletal
Uterus
Cardiovascular
Heme
Pulmonary
Renal
Endocrine
Gastrointestinal

PPx:

- Preconception folate supplementation
- Group B strep screening
- HIV/syphilis screening at 8 weeks
- Glucose tolerance test at 28 weeks
- Blood pressure (preeclampsia)
- Iron and multivitamin supplementation

MoD: Sperm meets egg to form zygote → implants into either in the endometrium (normal) or outside the endometrium (ectopic). Do NOT memorize stages of embryogenesis (e.g., what week gastrulation occurs, etc.) for the Ob/Gyn shelf.

Dx:

1. Beta-hCG blood or urine tests
2. Transvaginal ultrasound to confirm placement in uterus
3. Fetal Doppler to assess heart rate

Tx/Mgmt:

1. Vaginal delivery (preferred)
2. C section if contraindications to vaginal delivery
3. D&C if cervix found to be open <20 weeks
4. Misoprostol/mifepristone for spontaneous and induced abortions
5. Oxytocin to stimulate contraction during and after delivery
6. Corticosteroids to help mature the lungs of preterm fetuses
7. Morphine or epidural anesthesia for pain control during delivery

Ethics in Obstetrics/Gynecology

Ethical scenarios on the Ob/Gyn shelf are difficult because they often involve the health of both the mother and fetus. Sometimes you will encounter patient scenarios when the mother has made a decision that has a high probability of harming the fetus (e.g., drug use). However, the major organizing principle behind ethical questions on the shelf is that the mother gets as much leeway as possible with her decisions if she has the medical capacity to make the decision. This aligns with the 2016 **American College of Obstetricians and Gynecologists** (ACOG) recommendations for ethical dilemmas in Ob/Gyn. Thus, in answering these questions, view the pregnant woman and fetus as "interconnected and interdependent," championed by Ali et al. in their review article "Ethical Issues in Maternal–Fetal Care Emergencies."

As a disclaimer, the actions recommended in the following scenarios do not reflect the belief of the authors. Rather, these are the answers as you will likely see on the NBME shelf exam. You do not necessarily have to agree with the philosophy behind these questions to answer them correctly for testing purposes:

1. Pregnant patient refuses to stop using substances during pregnancy (e.g., alcohol, tobacco, cocaine, heroin):

   Action: Ask why, be respectful, recognize that the patient and fetus are interconnected, and offer resources for support if adverse events affect the fetus.

   Avoid: Coercion to force patient to stop using substances, punitive action, or scolding patient.

2. Pregnant patient refuses to take folate supplementation even though prior pregnancy led to a neural tube defect:

   Action: Ask why, be respectful, recognize that the patient and fetus are interconnected, offer resources for support if adverse events affect the fetus.

   Avoid: Coercion to force patient to stop using substances, punitive action, or scolding patient.

3. Pregnant patient at risk for shoulder dystocia refuses C section and desires a vaginal birth:

   Action: Respect decision, allow patient to proceed with a natural birth.

   Avoid: Court injunction for C-section.

4. Postpartum patient expresses a desire to kill her newborn:

   Action: Admit to hospital, assess and treat for postpartum psychosis and depression.

   Avoid: Normalizing the patient's thoughts and not taking the threat seriously.

5. Pregnant patient finds out that the fetus has Down syndrome and wishes to terminate the pregnancy within the legal time frame:

   Action: Respect patient decision.

   Avoid: Arguing for delivery of fetus at a viable gestational age, ideological or political confrontation.

6. Pregnant patient whose fetus becomes brain dead following traumatic injury:

   Action: Determine gestational age of fetus and viability, consult with significant other or next of kin, decide how to proceed based on discussions with family.

   Avoid: Making a decision without consultation with spouse, significant other, closest of kin.

ACOG Summary of ethical recommendations

Other ethical scenarios you've seen? Disagree with our answers? Email us at team@gunnergoggles.com.

7. Case of a pregnant Jehovah's Witness who is involved in a traumatic injury and needs a blood transfusion, which would save the lives of both mother and fetus:

Action: Determine if patient meets criteria for not needing informed consent (e.g., legally incompetent, implied consent in emergency with no ability for communication, patient waived right to informed consent).

Avoid: Giving blood if patient does not give consent and does not meet one of the exceptions.

GUNNER PRACTICE

1. A 30-year-old woman presents to the physician complaining of amenorrhea. She states that she has not had a menstrual cycle for the past 7 weeks and has noticed that she has to urinate more frequently. Her menstrual periods have come once every 35 days and are associated with a moderate amount of cramping that sometimes makes her grimace. She is sexually active with her male partner of 6 months and uses condoms occasionally. She has a history of *Chlamydia*, two episodes, which were treated with azithromycin. Her surgical history is notable for an appendectomy when she was 15. Her vitals are 100/60 mm Hg, 99°F, 90 bpm, 15 RR. On physical exam, there is no tenderness to palpation. Her uterus is slightly enlarged. She has not had a Pap smear since she was 21 years old. What is the best next step in management?
   A. Urinalysis and urine culture
   B. Beta-hCG
   C. Urine drug screen
   D. Luteinizing hormone and follicle-stimulating hormone levels
   E. Pap smear

2. A 21-year-old woman, gravida 1, para 1, comes to clinic with a positive home pregnancy test. Her last menstrual period that she can remember was 2 months earlier. She smokes 1 or 2 cigarettes a day and drinks a glass of wine with dinner once or twice a week. She has a healthy 2-year-old daughter. Her vital signs are 100/60 mm Hg, 98.6°F, 85 bpm, 12 RR. When counseled about the adverse effects of her tobacco and alcohol use on fetal development, she does not appear to be interested and states that she plans to continue her substance use. What is the most appropriate thing to say to the patient?

A. "I respect your lifestyle decisions. Given that your previous child did not experience any adverse developmental effects, I am less concerned about the effects of your tobacco and alcohol use on your current pregnancy."

B. "I respect your lifestyle decisions. Given that your tobacco and alcohol use is minimal, I am less concerned about the potential effects on your unborn child."

C. "I can offer you free resources discussing the dangers of substance use. However, I will have to call Child Protective Services if you choose to continue using substances that may cause significant medical harm to your unborn child."

D. "Using tobacco and drinking alcohol during pregnancy is extremely irresponsible behavior. How could you choose to harm your baby like this? You should be ashamed of risking the life of your unborn child."

E. "Your body and your baby's well-being are interconnected. May I ask why you choose to continue your tobacco and alcohol use?"

ANSWERS: What Would Gunner Jess/Jim Do?

1. WWGJD? A 30-year-old woman presents to the physician complaining of amenorrhea. She states that she has not had a menstrual cycle since 7 weeks ago and has noticed that she has to urinate more frequently. Her menstrual periods have come once every 35 days and are associated with a moderate amount of cramping that makes her grimace at work. She is sexually active with her partner of 6 months and uses condoms occasionally. She has a history of two episodes of chlamydia that were treated with azithromycin. Her surgical history is notable for an appendectomy when she was 15. Her vitals are 100/60 mm Hg, 99°F, 90, 15 RR. On physical exam, there is no tenderness to palpation. Her uterus is slightly enlarged. She has not had a Pap smear since she was 21 years old. What is the best next step in management?

Answer: B. Beta-hCG

Explanation: For the purposes of the Ob/Gyn shelf, the first test to order for any woman of childbearing age who presents with pelvic pain, abdominal discomfort, or amenorrhea is a pregnancy test. Patients who have systemic signs and symptoms of pregnancy, such as increased urinary frequency, should be evaluated for pregnancy as well. To answer this question quickly, recognize that this is amenorrhea in a woman of childbearing age, read the last sentence of the question stem, and feel confident in answering B. The content in the middle of the question is designed to confuse you and would not offer a better explanation of the amenorrhea.

A. Urinalysis and urine culture → Incorrect. Although the patient presents with urinary urgency, she does not complain of any other urinary symptoms, such as dysuria or hematuria. In addition, a UTI would not cause amenorrhea directly.

C. Urine drug screen → Incorrect. There are certain drugs and medications that can alter a patient's menstrual cycle, including hormonal treatments themselves. However, pregnancy in a woman of childbearing age must first be ruled out.

D. Luteinizing hormone and follicle-stimulating hormone levels → Incorrect. Certain disorders such as Turner syndrome can lead to amenorrhea. FSH and LH levels often help narrow down the amenorrhea differential. However, levels of pituitary hormones are for the most part obtained only after more common causes are ruled out.

    E. Pap smear → Incorrect. Although she is due for a Pap test, testing for cervical cancer as the next step would not be the appropriate management for a female of childbearing age presenting with amenorrhea.

2. WWGJD? A 21-year-old, gravida 1, para 1, woman comes to clinic with a positive home pregnancy test. Her last menstrual period that she can remember was 2 months ago. She smokes 1–2 cigarettes per day and drinks a glass of wine a night with dinner 1–2 times per week. She has a healthy 2-year-old daughter. Her vital signs are 100/60 mm Hg, 98.6°F, 85 bpm, 12 RR. When counseled about the adverse effects of her tobacco and alcohol use on fetal development, the patient does not appear interested in the subject and states that she plans to continue her substance use. What is the most appropriate thing to say to the patient?

Answer: E. "Your body and your baby's well-being are interconnected. May I ask why you choose to continue your tobacco and alcohol use?"

    Explanation: Ask why, be respectful, recognize that the patient and fetus are interconnected, offer resources for support if adverse events affect the fetus. Avoid coercion (forcing the patient to stop using substances), punitive action, or scolding.

    A. "I respect your lifestyle decisions. Given that your previous child did not experience any adverse developmental effects, I am less concerned about the effects of your tobacco and alcohol use on your current pregnancy." → Incorrect. According to current guidelines, there is no safe level of alcohol or tobacco usage during pregnancy. A previous healthy pregnancy does not change this fact.

    B. "I respect your lifestyle decisions. Given that your tobacco and alcohol use are minimal, I am less concerned about the potential effects on your unborn child." → Incorrect. According to current guidelines, there is no safe level of alcohol or tobacco usage during pregnancy.

    C. "I can offer you free resources discussing the dangers of substance use. However, I will have to call Child Protective Services if you choose to continue using substances which may cause significant medical harm to your unborn child." → Incorrect. Do not threaten the patient.

D. "Using tobacco and drinking alcohol during pregnancy is extremely irresponsible behavior. How could you choose to harm your baby like this? You should be ashamed of risking the life of your unborn child." → Incorrect. Do not scold the patient. This is disrespectful and may cause the patient to be less open and honest with you.

Breast Pathologies

Drake Lebrun, Rebecca W. Gao, Hao-Hua Wu, Leo Wang, and Holly W. Cummings

Introduction

Disorders of the breast are very high-yield. These include infectious and inflammatory conditions as well as benign and malignant neoplasms.

One of the most important organizing principles of this chapter is to understand the buzz words for common chief complaints, such as nipple discharge or breast masses. For example, for a question on nipple discharge, you need to know that different colors of discharge are associated with specific conditions: **straw-colored discharge** that varies cyclically is likely due to fibrocystic change, **purulent discharge** is likely due to a breast abscess, and **bloody discharge** is either due to intraductal papilloma or papillary carcinoma.

This chapter is divided into three main sections: (1) Infectious, Immunologic, and Inflammatory Disorders; (2) Benign Neoplasms or Masses; (3) Malignant Neoplasms; and (4) Gunner Practice. As always, each disease process is presented in the context of the four physician tasks that the shelf exam will test you on: (1) prophylactic management (PPx), (2) mechanism of disease (MoD), (3) diagnostic steps (Dx), and (4) treatment/management steps (Tx/Mgmt).

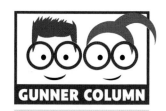

GUNNER COLUMN

Breast Disorders

Infectious, Immunologic, and Inflammatory Disorders

Mastitis

Buzz Words: Focal breast pain + breast erythema + nipple cracking + variations in temperature from one part of breast to another + infectious symptoms (fever, malaise, myalgias)

Clinical Presentation: A 30-year-old female breastfeeding her newborn complains of pain in her right breast without discharge and a fever for 2 days. On exam, the area of the right breast around the areola is tender and erythematous (Fig. 3.1).

PPx: N/A

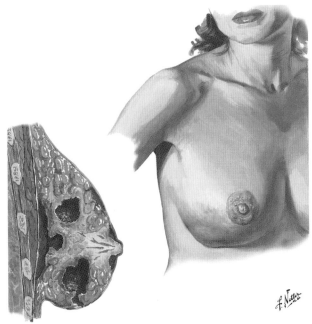

FIG. 3.1 Lactational mastitis.

MoD: Bacteria (most commonly *Staphylococcus aureus*) enter the breast via small cracks in the skin caused by breast-feeding, leading to a superficial infection of breast tissue.

Dx:
1. Physical exam revealing a tender, erythematous breast
2. Elevated WBC count

Tx/Mgmt:
1. Oral antistaphylococcal antibiotics are required. Dicloxacillin or cephalexin are first-line. Trimethoprim-sulfamethoxazole (TMP-SMX) is indicated if patient is at risk for methicillin-resistant *Staphylococcus aureus* (MRSA).
2. If unresponsive to oral antibiotics: IV antibiotics.
3. If unresponsive to IV antibiotics, suspect abscess, which requires surgical treatment.

Breast Abscess

Buzz Words: Painful, palpable, fluctuant breast mass + **purulent nipple discharge** + skin erythema + infectious symptoms (fever, malaise, myalgias)

Clinical Presentation: A 28-year-old woman who is breast-feeding her newborn has had left breast pain and a fever for a week. Over the last 2 days, she began having purulent yellow nipple discharge and increased swelling of her left breast.

PPx: Can be prevented by timely and appropriate treatment of mastitis and continued breastfeeding with the affected breast.

MoD: Progression of a superficial infection of breast tissue → localized collection of pus and associated tissue destruction

Dx:

1. Physical exam reveals **a warm, tender, fluctuant breast mass with associated purulent nipple discharge**
2. Elevated WBC
3. Ultrasound to localize mass

Tx/Mgmt:

1. Ultrasound-guided needle aspiration of abscess until no collection remains
2. If overlying skin is destroyed or if abscess is unresponsive to aspiration, incision and drainage

Fat Necrosis

Buzz Words: Pain **following trauma to breast** + skin retraction + spiculated calcifications on mammography

Clinical Presentation: A 35-year-old woman plays baseball regularly. On her most recent mammogram, the radiologist noted spiculated calcifications. Her risk factors include **pendulous breasts** and a **recent history of breast surgery.**

PPx: N/A

MoD: Trauma disrupts fatty breast tissue → fat cells undergo necrosis → release of cytokines incites a localized inflammatory response. Eventually reparative fibrosis walls off and replaces the area of fat necrosis.

Dx:

1. Implied history of trauma
2. Mammography: demonstrates ill-defined, irregular spiculated calcifications (Fig. 3.2)

Tx/Mgmt:

1. Reassurance and observation
2. Excision is unnecessary as there is no increased risk of breast cancer

Benign Neoplasms or Masses

Solitary Breast Cyst

Buzz Words: Small rounded or oval fluid-filled sac + nontender + smooth borders

Clinical Presentation: Often detected on routine breast exams. Should be on the differential for breast masses in premenopausal women.

QUICK TIPS

Pendulous breasts = deflated breast tissue, often with nipple pointing downward.

QUICK TIPS

Fat necrosis is caused by trauma to the breast, but patients may not recall or report any injury to the breast.

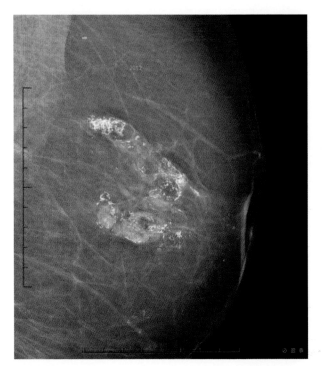

FIG. 3.2 Mammogram of a patient with fat necrosis demonstrating spiculated calcifications. (From https://radiopaedia.org/articles/fat-necrosis-breast-2.)

PPx: N/A

MoD: Lobule in the terminal grows into a fluid-filled mass.

Dx:

1. All palpable breast masses should be evaluated with:
   - Physical exam
   - Ultrasound and fine-needle aspiration (FNA)
   - Mammography

Tx/Mgmt:

1. Reassurance and observation; most cysts will resolve spontaneously
2. Drainage of fluid can be performed if the cyst enlarges or becomes painful

Fibrocystic Change

Buzz Words: Multiple painful bilateral breast masses + straw-colored nipple discharge + fluctuation in size and severity with menstrual cycle

Clinical Presentation: A young female (20s–30s) has a breast mass on routine physical exam. She notes that the mass enlarges and become tender cyclically with her periods.

PPx: None

MoD: Exaggerated response of breast tissue to physiologic hormonal changes during menstrual cycle

Dx:
1. History and physical exam
2. FNA of fluid
3. Mammogram

Tx/Mgmt:
1. Oral contraceptive pills
2. Danazol (androgen agonist), bromocriptine (dopamine agonist), and/or tamoxifen (selective estrogen antagonist in the breast) may be used in severe cases if OCPs are ineffective
3. Nonsteroidal anti-inflammatory drugs for pain control

Fibroadenoma

Buzz Words: Firm, rubbery, nontender round mass + freely movable + well-circumscribed + often solitary and unilateral + *no* fluctuation in size with menstrual cycle + slow or no growth (vs. phyllodes tumors, which grow rapidly)

Clinical Presentation: A young female (late teens to 20s) was found to have a breast mass on routine exam. The mass is firm, rubbery, and nontender to palpation. She has not noticed any change in the size of the mass over the past year.

PPx: N/A

MoD: Benign proliferation of breast epithelium and stroma

Dx:
1. Physical exam
2. Mammogram to visualize lesion (Fig. 3.3)
3. Ultrasound to differentiate solid vs. cystic components + FNA

Tx/Mgmt:
1. If asymptomatic: Observation and reassurance. Most fibroadenomas will be reabsorbed.
2. If mass enlarges or is persistent for more than 3 months, excisional biopsy.
3. If mass is very large (>5 cm), core needle biopsy to rule out cystosarcoma phyllodes.

Phyllodes Tumor (Cystosarcoma Phyllodes)

Buzz Words: Very large (>6 cm) nontender mass + warm erythematous skin overlying mass + freely movable + well circumscribed + rapid growth

Clinical Presentation: A female (40s–50s) complains of a breast mass, which is growing rapidly in size at a constant rate. Its size does not vary with her menstrual cycle, and there is no nipple discharge.

Disorders of the breast

QUICK TIPS

Fibrocystic change usually fluctuates with the menstrual cycle. Fibroadenomas do not.

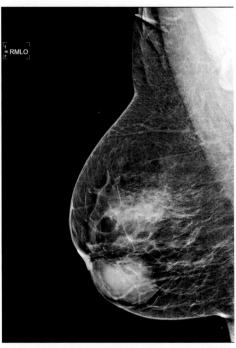

FIG. 3.3 Mammogram of a fibroadenoma, demonstrating a small well-circumscribed solid lesion. (From https://radiopaedia.org/cases/fibroadenoma-of-the-breast-1.)

PPx: N/A

MoD: Benign proliferation of breast epithelium and stroma that may contain malignant cells

Dx:

1. Mammogram to visualize lesion
2. Ultrasound to differentiate solid vs. cystic components
3. **Core-needle biopsy** to rule out underlying aggressive malignancy

Tx/Mgmt: Wide local excision owing to:

1. High rate of local recurrence with simple excision and
2. 10% of phyllodes tumors contain malignant cells

Intraductal Papilloma

Buzz Words: Unilateral bloody or serosanguinous nipple discharge

Clinical Presentation: A female (20s–40s) complains of unilateral bloody nipple discharge. There are no breast masses on physical exam.

PPx: N/A

MoD: Benign growth of epithelial lining (papilloma) arises within the lactiferous ducts (intraductal). Large papillomas blocks duct, causing infarction → bloody discharge.

TABLE 3.1 Breast Neoplasms

	Description	Classic Presentation	Treatment
Lobular carcinoma in situ (LCIS)	**Noninvasive** proliferation of malignant epithelial cells in breast **lobules**	Asymptomatic Incidental finding on biopsy for an unrelated indication	Observe Selective estrogen-receptor modifiers
Ductal carcinoma in Situ (DCIS)	**Noninvasive** proliferation of malignant epithelial cells in breast **ducts**	Asymptomatic Found on screening mammography showing clustered microcalcifications	Lumpectomy + radiation therapy Simple mastectomy for extensive multicentric lesions
Invasive cancer		Ill-defined, fixed breast mass Irregular asymmetric mass with spiculations and architectural distortion on imaging	Lumpectomy + radiation therapy Simple mastectomy for larger lesions Radical mastectomy for disease with axillary node involvement
Lobular carcinoma	Invasive proliferation of malignant epithelial cells in breast **lobules**	Less common than ductal carcinoma Frequently bilateral	
Ductal carcinoma	Invasive proliferation of malignant epithelial cells in breast **ducts**	More common that lobular carcinoma	

Dx:
1. Cytology of discharge to rule out invasive papillary cancer.
2. Mammogram to rule out other lesions. Mammogram will not show the papilloma because of its small size.

Tx/Mgmt:
1. Surgical excision of involved duct

Malignant Neoplasms

Breast Cancer

Buzz Words: Irregular fixed breast mass + asymmetric + architectural distortion + retraction of overlying skin and/ or nipple + "orange peel" skin texture (peau d'orange) + eczematous lesion of nipple/areola + palpable axillary lymph nodes

See Table 3.1 for specific buzz words for each type of cancer.

Clinical Presentation: Most commonly seen in postmenopausal females. Key elements of the history to watch out for:
- History of ductal carcinoma in situ (DCIS) or lobular carcinoma in situ (LCIS)

> **QUICK TIPS**
> The two important causes of bloody nipple discharge are intraductal papilloma (benign) and papillary breast cancer (malignant).

TABLE 3.2 Surgical and Adjuvant Treatment Options for Breast Cancer

	Description	Indications
Lumpectomy	Segmental resection of lesion with margins, leaving most of breast tissue and overlying skin intact	Small breast neoplasms located away from the nipple/areolar complex in a larger breast
Simple mastectomy	Removal of all breast tissue and overlying skin, leaving axillary contents intact	Large breast neoplasms near the nipple/areolar complex in a large breast; breast neoplasms that occupy most of a small breast
Radical mastectomy	Removal of all breast tissue, overlying skin, axillary contents, and pectoralis minor muscle	Breast neoplasms with lymphatic spread
Sentinel lymph node biopsy	Sentinel lymph node is identified by radioactive tracer injected near the tumor and is then removed and biopsied to assess for metastasis	Lumpectomies and simple mastectomies

- Increased lifetime estrogen exposure due to younger age at menarche, nulliparity, older age of first live birth, older age at menopause, obesity, or long-term (>5 years) use of hormone-replacement therapy
- Prior exposure to ionizing radiation (e.g., treatment of Hodgkin lymphoma during childhood)
- Family history of gynecologic malignancies
- First-degree relatives with breast cancer. Risk increases with number of first-degree relatives and early age at time of diagnosis.
- *BRCA1/BRCA2* genes are associated with bilateral premenopausal breast cancer and ovarian cancer.

PPx
- ACOG: Annual mammograms starting at age 40
- U.S. Preventive Services Task Force (USPTF): Biennial mammograms from age 50 to 74
- American Cancer Society: Annual mammograms from age 45 to 54, then annual or biennial for as long as woman is in good health
- Prophylactic mastectomy for *BRCA*-positive

MoD: N/A

Dx:
1. Screening mammography
2. Core needle biopsy or FNA for definitive diagnosis
3. Staging workup for metastatic disease

Tx/Mgmt:
1. See Tables 3.1 and 3.2

QUICK TIPS

Obesity increases lifetime estrogen exposure because excess adipose tissue converts androgens into estrogens.

Inflammatory Breast Carcinoma

Buzz Words: Breast dimpling + failed antibiotic treatment for mastitis

Clinical Presentation: A 39-year-old woman was prescribed antibiotics for mastitis 3 weeks earlier. She has adhered to her antibiotic regimen but her right breast is increasingly tender, erythematous, and diffusely swollen. She now has dimpling of her breast and axillary lymphadenopathy.

PPx: N/A

MoD: None

Tx/Mgmt:

1. An aggressive cancer that is often metastatic on initial presentation
2. Treat with chemoradiation

Paget Disease of the Breast

Buzz Words: Eczema (scaling, crusting, ulceration) of the nipple/areolar complex + unilateral + malignant intraepithelial cells (Paget cells) + concurrent underlying breast cancer

Clinical Presentation: A female presents with erythema, scaling, and crusting surrounding her left nipple. She is not breastfeeding.

PPx: N/A

MoD: Malignant cells invade the epidermis of the nipple → inflammation of the nipple → spread to areola → eczematous changes of the nipple/areolar complex

Dx:

1. You must remember to evaluate for breast cancer because Paget disease of the breast is almost always associated with an underlying neoplasm.
   • Diagnostic biopsy of skin demonstrating presence of intraepithelial adenocarcinoma cells (Paget cells) within the nipple
   • Mammography to identify the breast mass

Tx/Mgmt:

1. Surgical resection of the lesion
2. The type of surgery and adjuvant therapy will depend on the stage of the concurrent underlying breast cancer (Fig. 3.4).

GUNNER PRACTICE

1. A 42-year-old female presents to her gynecologist for a lump in her left breast. She states that she first noticed the lump 2 months earlier. The lump has grown rapidly, which prompted this visit. It is firm, nontender, and not associated with nipple discharge. She denies

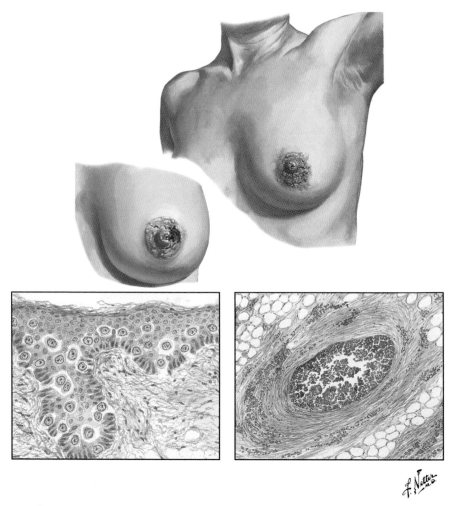

FIG. 3.4 Classic physical exam findings with Paget disease (scaling, crusting, ulceration near the nipple/areolar complex).

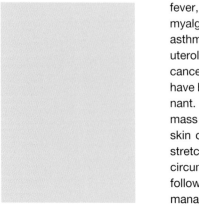

fever, chills, chest wall tenderness, shortness of breath, myalgias, or muscle weakness. She has a history of asthma that is well controlled with intermittent albuterol. She has no family history of breast or ovarian cancer. Menarche occurred at age 12 and her periods have been regular since then. She has never been pregnant. Examination reveals a large, firm, freely movable mass in the upper outer quadrant of the left breast. The skin overlying the mass appears shiny and somewhat stretched. A mammogram demonstrates a 6-cm well-circumscribed mass with smooth margins. Which of the following is the most appropriate next best step in the management of this patient?

A. Fine-needle aspiration
B. Magnetic resonance imaging
C. Reassurance and observation
D. Lumpectomy followed by adjuvant radiation therapy
E. Core needle biopsy

2. A 61-year-old woman presents to her gynecologist for a red rash on her left breast. She reports that the rash started 6 months earlier and has been associated with persistent itchiness and crusting despite multiple treatments with over-the-counter moisturizing creams. She denies nipple discharge or breast pain. She denies fever, chills, weight loss, or change in appetite. She has a history of hypertension and hyperlipidemia, which are well controlled. Physical exam is notable for a red crusty ulcerative lesion approximately 3 cm in diameter overlying the left nipple and areola. In addition to performing a skin biopsy of the lesion, what other step is most appropriate in the management of this patient?

A. Leuprolide
B. Breast ultrasound
C. Mammogram
D. Topical steroid
E. Wide local excision of the nipple/areolar complex

ANSWERS: What Would Gunner Jess/Jim Do?

1. **WWGJD?** A 42-year-old female presents to her gynecologist for a lump in her left breast. She states that she first noticed the lump 2 months ago. The lump has grown rapidly in size since she first noticed it, which prompted her to visit her gynecologist. The lump is firm, nontender, and not associated with nipple discharge. She denies fever, chills, chest wall tenderness, shortness of breath, myalgias, or muscle weakness. She has a history of asthma that is well controlled with intermittent albuterol. She has no family history of breast or ovarian cancer. Menarche occurred at age 12 and her periods have been regular since then. She has never been pregnant. Examination reveals a large, firm, freely moveable mass in the upper outer quadrant of the patient's left breast. The skin overlying the mass appears shiny and somewhat stretched. A mammogram demonstrates a large 6-cm well-circumscribed mass with smooth margins. Which of the following is the most appropriate next best step in the management of this patient?

Answer: E. Core needle biopsy

Explanation: This patient in her early 40s presents with a rapidly growing freely movable well-circumscribed breast mass. This is most consistent with **cystosarcoma phyllodes (phyllodes tumor).** These tumors are proliferations of epithelial and stromal breast tissue, similar to fibroadenomas. However, unlike fibroadenomas, phyllodes tumors often occur in women in their 30s and 40s, are larger, grow more rapidly, and may harbor malignant cells. Core needle biopsy is the preferred method of definitive pathologic diagnosis for cystosarcoma phyllodes after initial imaging.

A. Fine-needle aspiration → incorrect. FNA has a high false-negative rate and is not appropriate for biopsy of potential phyllodes tumors. Core needle biopsy is the preferred method for making a pathologic diagnosis.

B. Magnetic resonance imaging → Incorrect. Although more advanced imaging modalities such as MRI may better characterize this mass, a pathologic diagnosis is required.

C. Reassurance and observation → Incorrect. Cystosarcoma phyllodes may harbor malignant cells; thus, tissue biopsy is required to confirm the diagnosis and rule out malignancy. Reassurance and observation would be appropriate if this mass were a smaller and less locally aggressive fibroadenoma.

D. Lumpectomy followed by adjuvant radiation therapy → Incorrect. A definitive tissue diagnosis is required before surgery is performed.

2. **WWGJD? A 61-year-old woman** presents to her gynecologist for a **red rash on her left breast.** She reports that the **rash started 6 months ago** and has been associated with **persistent itchiness and crusting** despite multiple treatments with over-the-counter moisturizing creams. She denies nipple discharge or breast pain. She denies fever, chills, weight loss, or change in appetite. She has a history of hypertension and hyperlipidemia, which are well controlled. Physical exam is notable for **a red crusty ulcerative lesion,** approximately 3 centimeters in diameter, overlying the left nipple and areola. In addition to performing a skin biopsy of the lesion, what other step is most appropriate in the management of this patient?

Answer: C. Mammogram

Explanation: This postmenopausal female presents with an eczematous lesion affecting the nipple, most consistent with **Paget disease of the breast.** This disease is frequently associated with a concurrent underlying breast neoplasm. In addition to skin biopsy to confirm the diagnosis of Paget disease, this patient should also undergo mammography to identify any potential underlying neoplasms.

A. Leuprolide → Incorrect. Leuprolide is a GnRH analogue that decreases levels of estrogen and testosterone. It is used to treat uterine fibroids and certain types of breast cancer. It is not used to treat Paget disease of the breast.

B. Breast ultrasound → Incorrect. Breast ultrasound may help to identify an underlying breast neoplasm; however, mammogram is more sensitive than ultrasound alone.

D. Topical steroid → Incorrect. Topical steroid is not an appropriate treatment for Paget disease of the breast.

E. Wide local excision of the nipple/areolar complex → Incorrect. A definitive tissue diagnosis is required before any surgery is performed.

Infections of the Female Reproductive System

Hao-Hua Wu, Rebecca W. Gao, Angela Ester Ugorets, Leo Wang, and Holly W. Cummings

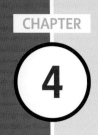

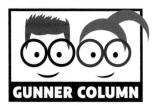

GUNNER COLUMN

Introduction

This is a high-yield chapter because many of the disorders are multidisciplinary, such as sexually transmitted infections (STIs). Expect to have at least five questions on these on exam day. The most high-yield STI is syphilis, also known as "the great imitator." Another important concept is Fitz-Hugh-Curtis syndrome, which is a perihepatitis that arises from *Chlamydia* and gonorrhea. For STIs, focus on buzz words and know the gold standard for diagnosis and treatment (e.g., RPR and VDRL to diagnose syphilis; doxycycline/ceftriaxone to treat *Chlamydia*/gonorrhea, respectively). Also, you must know how to differentiate painful ulcers (e.g., herpes and chancroid) from painless ulcers (e.g., syphilis and granuloma inguinale).

Infectious, Immunologic, and Inflammatory Disorders

Bacterial Vaginosis

Buzz Words: White/gray thin discharge + **clue cells** + pH >4.5 + fishy odor with KOH

Clinical Presentation: A reproductive-age woman presents with white-gray vaginal discharge and a fishy odor, which worsens after sexual intercourse. Risk factors include frequent sexual intercourse and vaginal douching, the most common cause of vaginitis.

PPx: Avoid vaginal douching, which alters normal vaginal flora.

MoD: Imbalance in normal vaginal bacteria leading to anaerobic bacteria proliferation, such as *Gardenella vaginalis*. This is NOT an STI.

Dx:
1. Vaginal discharge with a pH > 4 (alkaline)
2. Clue cells under the microscope
3. Positive whiff test (fishy odor when adding KOH to sample of discharge)

Tx/Mgmt:
1. Metronidazole or clindamycin
2. Treatment is indicated for pregnant women because untreated BV can cause preterm birth.

QUICK TIPS

Warn your patient to not drink alcohol while taking metronidazole as this can cause a disulfram-like reaction (flushing, nausea).

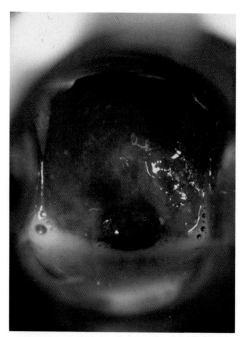

FIG. 4.1 Strawberry cervix on pelvic exam. (From http://www.medicinejournal.co.uk/action/showFullTextImages?pii=S1357-3039%2810%2900074-5.)

Trichomonas

Buzz Words: Gray, yellow, green discharge + strawberry (red petichiae) cervix + pH >4.5 + corkscrew motility

Clinical Presentation: A woman with multiple sexual partners and minimal use of protection presents with yellow-green vaginal discharge with a musty odor. On pelvic exam, she has an inflamed cervix with red petechiae ("strawberry cervix") (Fig. 4.1).

PPx
- Condom usage
- Treat sexual partner with metronidazole

MoD: *Trichomonas vaginalis* is a sexually transmitted protozoan.

Dx:
1. Visualization of flagellated protozoa under microscope ("swimming" across the slide, sometimes called "corkscrew" or "quivering" motility) (Fig. 4.2).
2. pH of vaginal discharge >4.5
3. Note: Most men and many women are asymptomatic.

Tx/Mgmt:
1. Metronidazole
2. Can treat during pregnancy, as untreated *T. vaginalis* is associated with premature birth and low birth weight.

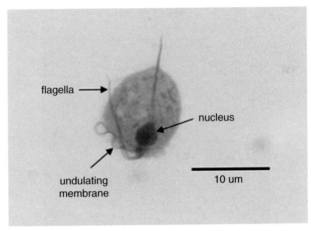

flagella

nucleus

undulating
membrane

10 um

FIG. 4.2 Protozoa with flagella on wet mount. (From http://faculty.
ccbcmd.edu/courses/bio141/lecguide/unit4/protozoa/tricho.html.)

Candidiasis

Buzz Words: Cottage-cheese/clumpy/curd-like discharge +
hyphae on KOH + pH <4.5

Clinical Presentation: Vaginal candidiasis, also known as a
yeast infection, is the second most common cause of
vaginitis. A common presentation: A female with diabetes presents with uncomfortable red, itchy vulva, and
thick, clumpy, white vaginal discharge. She reports
pain on urination and with sexual intercourse. Risk factors include recent antibiotics use, which may kill off
normal vaginal bacteria and allow the yeast to flour-
ish, and diabetes, as these patients spill glucose into
their urine, which leads to better conditions for yeast
to grow.

PPx: Tighter control of blood glucose level in diabetics,
avoidance of unnecessary antibiotic usage

MoD: Overgrowth of normal vaginal yeast, *Candida albi-
cans.* This is NOT an STI.

Dx:

1. Thick white cottage cheese–like vaginal discharge
   with a pH <4.5 (different from bacterial vaginosis and
   trichomoniasis)
2. Branching hyphae under the microscope with KOH
   prep
3. Negative whiff test

Tx/Mgmt:

1. Antifungal agents ("-azole"), such as oral fluconazole
   or vaginal butoconazole

gg AR

Differentiating BV, Trich,
Candidiasis

Bartholin Gland Cyst

Definition: A common vulvar mass that forms due to cystic dilation of an obstructed Bartholin gland duct.

Buzz Words: Cystic vulvar mass + 4-o'clock or 8-o'clock position

Clinical Presentation: A painless vulvar mass, often asymptomatic but occasionally causing discomfort due to its size

PPx: N/A

MoD: Bartholin glands function to lubricate the vagina and vulva by producing mucous secretions. These ducts open into the vulvar vestibule at 4- and 8-o'clock positions on each side of the vagina and can become obstructed, forming a cyst or, if infected, an abscess.

Dx:

1. Clinical diagnosis of finding a soft, painless vulvar mass at the site of a Bartholin gland duct

Tx/Mgmt:

1. No treatment is required for asymptomatic Bartholin cysts.
2. If the cyst is painful, fluctuant, or swollen, it is more likely to be a Bartholin gland abscess and will require incision and drainage followed by either marsupialization or placement of a catheter to prevent recurrence.

Urinary Tract Infection (Cystitis)

Buzz Words: Catheter + dysuria (burning on urination) + urinary frequency/urgency + suprapubic tenderness

Clinical Presentation: UTIs are much more prevalent in women than in men. Risk factors include pregnancy, indwelling catheters, diabetes (also increases the risk of ascension to kidneys), and structural abnormalities.

PPx: Appropriate hygiene

MoD: Usually an ascending infection from the urethra

Common pathogens:

- *Escherichia coli*—most common cause overall
- *Staphylococcus saprophyticus*—common in sexually active young women
- *Enterococcus, Klebsiella, Proteus, Pseudomonas, Enterobacter*—catheter-associated UTIs

Dx:

1. Urine dipstick test shows presence of
2. High levels of white blood cells (WBCs):
   - Leukocyte esterase—indicates WBCs in urine (pyuria)
   - Nitrite—positive for gram-negative bacteria; negative nitrites on dipstick do NOT exclude cystitis.

Tx/Mgmt:

1. Asymptomatic—two successive positive cultures with $>10^5$ colony-forming units (CFUs); treated only if patient is pregnant or going to have urologic surgery.
2. Uncomplicated; empiric treatment is appropriate:
   - Oral **TMP/SMX** is first-line.
   - Nitrofurantoin, fosfomycin, or fluoroquinolones are second-line.

Chlamydia

Buzz Words: <24 years old + purulent discharge + dysuria → chlamydial urethritis

Clinical Presentation: *Chlamydia* is the most common bacterial STI and is often asymptomatic. Presents as purulent discharge, abnormal bleeding, and dysuria in a reproductive-age female. It is a leading cause of infertility due to pelvic inflammatory disease (PID) and tubal scarring. It can cause cervicitis, PID, tubo-ovarian abscess, Fitz-Hugh–Curtis syndrome, and infertility.

PPx: Abstinence, condoms

MoD: Intracellular bacteria, *C. trachomatis*

Dx:

1. Nucleic acid amplification test (NAAT)
2. Gram stain; should be negative because chlamydial infection is intracellular.

Tx/Mgmt:

1. Azithromycin or doxycycline

Gonorrhea

Buzz Words: Migratory polyarthritis + endocarditis + rash → disseminated gonorrhea

Clinical Presentation: Gonorrhea is one of the most common STIs and can cause cervicitis, PID, tubo-ovarian abscess, Fitz-Hugh–Curtis syndrome, and infertility as well. It is often asymptomatic.

PPx: Abstinence, condoms

MoD: Sexual transmission of *Neisseria gonorrhoeae*

Dx:

1. Test sexually active patients regularly:
   - NAAT
   - Gram stain; should be positive for **gram-negative diplococci.**

Tx/Mgmt:

1. Ceftriaxone (for the gonorrhea) + azithromycin (for the concomitant chlamydial infection).
2. Hospitalize if infection is disseminated.

Pelvic Inflammatory Disease

Buzz Words: **Cervical motion tenderness** + chandelier sign

Clinical Presentation: Females may complain of low abdominal pain, cramps, fever, and cervical motion tenderness on exam. Patients can have so much pain that they "jump to the chandelier" when the examiner is performing a pelvic exam and feeling the patient's cervix ("chandelier sign"). Because PID is often a result of an untreated STI, risk factors include having multiple sexual partners and not using condoms. Complications of untreated PID include adhesions, causing infertility.

PPx: Test new sexual partners, usage of condoms, treat of STIs before they progress to PID.

MoD: PID occurs when an infection of the vagina ascends to the cervix, uterus, fallopian tubes, ovaries, or further into the pelvis. The most common causes are *N. gonorrhea* and *C. trachomatis.*

Dx:

1. Clinical diagnosis
2. Laparoscopy (definitive diagnosis)

Tx/Mgmt:

1. If patient is vomiting and unable to tolerate eating/ drinking, is febrile, or is unlikely to follow-up, inpatient treatment with IV ceftriaxone or cefoxitin or cefotetan + doxycycline.
2. Outpatient: clindamycin + gentamicin

Fitz-Hugh–Curtis Syndrome

Buzz Words: Violin-string adhesions on liver

Clinical Presentation: A reproductive-age female presents with **severe right-upper-quadrant (RUQ) pain** worsened by coughing. She has a fever and is sexually active with multiple partners.

PPx: Risk factors and prevention are the same as those for PID, as this is a result of untreated PID.

MoD: When PID is not treated, the infection can spread into the peritoneum and cause perihepatitis (inflammation of the liver capsule) and adhesions between the liver capsule (the Glison capsule) and the parietal peritoneum lining the abdominal wall and diaphragm. The adhesions are classically described as "violin-string adhesions." This causes RUQ pain and may cause systemic symptoms of infection. The patient may not have any other symptoms of PID, but the causative bacteria are almost always *N. gonorrheae* or *C. trachomatis.*

QUICK TIPS

Patients with suspected PID on clinical exam should be treated with antibiotics owing to the risk of infertility, tubo-ovarian abscess, or Fitz-Hugh-Curtis syndrome with untreated PID.

AR

Fitz-Hugh-Curtis Syndrome

Dx:
1. Clinical diagnosis of RUQ pain and positive cervical culture of *N. gonorrhea* or *C. trachomatis*.
2. Symptoms of PID such as cervical motion tenderness are NOT necessary for a diagnosis of Fitz-Hugh–Curtis syndrome.

Tx/Mgmt:
1. Antibiotics for appropriate organisms
2. The patient may also require laparoscopy to cut adhesions between the Glison capsule and surrounding peritoneum.

Human Papillomavirus

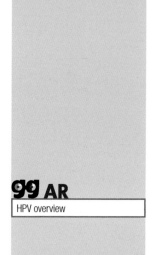

gg AR
HPV overview

Buzz Words: Genital warts + cervical dysplasia + ovarian or anal cancer

Clinical Presentation: One of the most common STIs is due to human papillomavirus (HPV), which has multiple strains. HPV 6 and HPV 11 are low-risk and causes condyloma acuminatum (genital warts). HPV 16, 18, 31, 33, and 45 are high-risk strains that can lead to cervical dysplasia and cancer.

PPx:
- Gardasil: quadrivalent vaccine indicated for women 11–26 years old
- Abstinence from sexual activity

MoD: Skin-skin contact

Dx:
1. Clinical presentation

Tx/Mgmt:
1. Podophyllin for relieving genital warts

Syphilis

gg AR
Syphilis stage

Buzz Words
- **Primary syphilis:** Sexually active + **painless ulcer** + lymphadenopathy + RPR-/VDRL-positive
- **Secondary syphilis:** Brown macular **rash on palms and soles** (copper-penny lesions) + condylomata lata + lymphadenopathy + constitutional symptoms (fever/myalgias/malaise) + painless ulcers
- **Tertiary syphilis:** Pupil constricts with accommodation but unreactive to light (**Argyll Robertson pupil**) + granulomas + broad-based ataxia due to **tabes dorsalis**) + inflammation of the aorta
- **Congenital syphilis:** newborn + **rhinitis** + hepatosplenomegaly + skin lesions + interstitial keratitis + **Hutchinson incisors** (smaller teeth, widely spaced,

with notches on biting surfaces) + saddle nose +
saber shins + deafness

Clinical Presentation: Syphilis is the most high-yield STI and one of the most commonly tested topics on the shelf because it has four different presentations: primary, secondary, tertiary, and congenital.

Syphilis will show up not only on your Ob/Gyn shelf but very likely on every other shelf as well. Thus the key is to recognize both buzz words and how to differentiate syphilis from diseases with similar presentations (e.g., vs. granuloma inguinale and lymphogranuloma venereum [LGV] for painless ulcers; vs. Rocky Mountain spotted fever and hand-foot-mouth disease; and from Coxsackie A virus for rash on palms/soles of foot). In addition, know that definitive diagnosis is made by dark-field microscopy and penicillin is used for treatment. Last, be mindful that congenital syphilis is unlikely to be tested on the Medicine shelf but is included here for the sake of completeness.

PPx: Barrier contraception

MoD: Syphilis is an STI caused by *Treponema pallidum*, a spirochete that disseminates infection widely throughout the body.

Dx:
1. RPR
2. VDRL (may be false-positive with lupus, rheumatic fever, and viral infections)
3. If VDRL-positive at 1:4 → progress to fluorescent treponemal antibody absorption test (FTA-ABS)
4. Definitive diagnosis = dark field microscopy
5. Test for concomitant HIV (and HBV if newborn)

Tx/Mgmt:
1. Penicillin
2. If patient is allergic to penicillin, desensitize by incremental doses of PO penicillin V

Granuloma Inguinale

Buzz Words: Red, beefy, smelly ulcers + **painless ulcers** + facial ulcers + **NO lymphadenopathy** + **Donovan bodies**

Clinical Presentation: Granuloma inguinale should be on the differential for any patient with painless ulcers.

PPx: Barrier contraception and testing of sexual partners

MoD: STI caused by *Klebsiella granulomatis*

Dx:
1. Culture; microscopic examination showing Donovan bodies

QUICK TIPS

Argyll Robertson pupils are also known as the "prostitute's pupil" because it accommodates but never reacts.

QUICK TIPS

Patients with syphilis can experience flu-like symptoms such as muscle ache and fever after taking antibiotics. This is known as Jarisch Hersheimer reaction and is 2/2 to toxin release by spriochetes.

QUICK TIPS

Granuloma inguinale vs. syphilis: Both have painless ulcers, but syphilis also has concomitant lymphadenopathy.

Tx/Mgmt:
1. Tetracycline drugs (e.g., doxycycline)
2. TMP/SMX
3. Azithromycin

Lymphogranuloma Venereum

Buzz Words: Painless ulcers + small, shallow ulcers (often asymptomatic) + matted lymph nodes (adjacent lymph nodes that become stuck together) + large, **painless,** fluctuant "buboes" + sinus tracts

Clinical Presentation: LGV should be on the differential for any patient with painless ulcers. The characteristic physical exam feature is the buboes, and it can occur in three stages:
1. An asymptomatic skin lesion appears.
2. Two weeks later, buboes (fluctuant masses) appear.
3. Scarring from inflammation may obstruct lymphatic vessels and cause swelling. Late-stage complications include pericarditis and arthralgias.

PPx: Barrier contraception and testing of sexual partners

MoD: LGV is an STI caused by *C. trachomatis* serovars L1-3, which are different from serotypes that cause vaginitis, conjunctivitis, and cervicitis. Unlike the others, L1-3 can invade lymph nodes.

Dx:
1. ELISA to look for antibodies to chlamydial endotoxin

Tx/Mgmt:
1. Tetracycline drugs (e.g., doxycycline)
2. Erythromycin
3. Surgical drainage of buboes

Chancroid

Buzz Words: Small **painful** papules present for 3–7 days followed by breakdown to shallow, soft, painful ulcers + ragged undetermined edges + red border + tender lymphadenopathy (LAD) + formation of swollen inflamed lymph node (bubo) with pus inside

Clinical Presentation: Chancroid is an STI caused by *Haemophilus ducreyi.* It is on the differential for painful genital lesions.

PPx: Barrier contraception and testing of sexual partners

MoD: Infection caused by *H. ducreyi*—gram-negative bacillus with rounded ends

Dx:
1. Clinical diagnosis
2. Culture (difficult to culture) or polymerase chain reaction (PCR)
3. Test for other STIs such as HIV and syphilis

QUICK TIPS

LGV vs. syphilis and granuloma inguinale: LGV has buboes and sinus tracts whereas the other two do not.

99 AR

Stages of LGV

99 AR

Painful and painless genital ulcers mnemonic

QUICK TIPS

- Chancroid vs. LGV: Chancroid buboes are **painful,** whereas LGV buboes are **painless.**
- Chancroid vs. HSV: Both are painful. Chancroid has associated buboes whereas HSV has only recurring, isolated painful lesions.

Tx/Mgmt:
1. Azithromycin
2. Ceftriaxone
3. Aspirate buboes

99 AR

Treatment of chancroid

GUNNER PRACTICE

1. A 17-year-old, gravida 0, para 0, girl presents to the doctor's office with a complaint of a foul odor. For the past week, she has noticed vaginal discharge and a foul odor that has negatively affected her sex life. She has been sexually active for 3 years and has had multiple partners. Her partners usually wear condoms but she takes oral contraceptives just in case. She has never tested positive for a sexually transmitted disease. Her vitals are 120/80 mm Hg, 75 bpm, 98.9°F, and 13 RR. Her pelvic exam is notable for a white, pungent discharge. Under the microscope, clue cells are visualized. What is the most appropriate treatment?
A. Azithromycin
B. Penicillin
C. Metronidazole
D. Itraconazole
E. Rifampin

ANSWER: What Would Gunner Jess/Jim Do?

1. WWGJD? A 17-year-old, gravida 0, para 0, girl presents to the doctor's office with a complaint of a **foul odor**. For the past week, she has noticed vaginal discharge and a foul odor that has negatively impacted her sexual activity. She has been sexually active for the past 3 years and has had multiple partners. Her partners usually wear condoms but she takes oral contraceptives just in case. She has never tested positive for a sexually transmitted disease. Her vitals are 120/80 mm Hg, 75 bpm, 98.9°F, and 13 RR. Her pelvic **exam is notable for white, pungent discharge. Under the microscope, clue cells are visualized. What is the most appropriate treatment?**

Answer: C. Metronidazole

Explanation: This patient has bacterial vaginosis, as evidenced by the foul odor, whitish vaginal discharge, and clue cells seen under the microscope. The treatment for BV is metronidazole. The most recognizable buzz word is "clue cells" which can refer only to BV on the Ob/Gyn shelf.

A. Azithromycin → Incorrect. Azithromycin can be used to treat *Chlamydia* but is not first-line for BV.

B. Penicillin → Incorrect. Penicillin can be used to treat syphilis but is not first-line for BV.

D. Itraconazole → Incorrect. Although a white discharge may sometimes connote a fungal infection, the clue cells point to bacterial vaginosis, which is caused by anaerobic lactobacilli.

E. Rifampin → Incorrect. Rifampin is an antibiotic used for tuberculosis therapy.

Neoplasms of the Ovary, Uterus, Cervix, Vagina, and Vulva

Esther Baranov, Rebecca W. Gao, Hao-Hua Wu, Leo Wang, and Holly W. Cummings

Introduction

Neoplasms of the gynecologic tract can be most easily triaged by their precancerous lesions and risk factors. Cervical, vaginal, and vulvar squamous cell carcinoma (SCC) are all mechanistically preceded by epithelial dysplasia caused by persistent human papillomavirus (HPV) infection. Therefore, they are associated with risk factors that lead to HPV infection (early coitus, multiple sexual partners, and sexually transmitted infections) or difficulty clearing the virus (immunosuppression, human immunodeficiency virus [HIV]). Endometrial cancer (EC) is preceded by atypical endometrial hyperplasia, which is associated with chronic exposure to high estrogen levels that are unopposed by progesterone. Thus, its risk factors often relate to excess estrogen, such as obesity, nulliparity, infertility, and polycystic ovarian syndrome (PCOS). Ovarian epithelial cancer, on the other hand, is associated with risk factors that lead to more numerous ovulatory cycles, such as early menarche, late menopause, nulliparity, and age.

Additionally, it is important to recognize presenting symptoms of gynecologic neoplasms. Many benign and malignant gynecologic neoplasms present with abnormal uterine bleeding (AUB) or postmenopausal bleeding (PMB), which are important clues that the patients are at risk for a gynecologic neoplasm. In other words, **postmenopausal bleeding is cancer until proven otherwise,** and **AUB in reproductive-aged women always warrants further testing**. An important scheme for systematically categorizing AUB is the PALM-COEIN (polyp, adenomyosis, leiomyoma, malignancy and hyperplasia, coagulopathy, ovulatory dysfunction, endometrial, iatrogenic, and not otherwise classified) system for nonpregnant, reproductive-aged women. Note that three of these categories are uterine masses.

This chapter is primarily divided in sections discussing each organ of the gynecological tract and then further subdivided into benign versus malignant etiologies. As always, each disease will be outlined by the four physician tasks

GUNNER COLUMN

MNEMONIC
PALM-COEIN system for classifying abnormal uterine bleeding (AUB) in non-pregnant reproductive-aged women:
Polyp (endometrial or endocervical polyps)
Adenomyosis
Leiomyoma (fibroids)
Malignancy/hyperplasia (endometrial hyperplasia or carcinoma)
Coagulopathy
Ovulatory dysfunction
Endometrial
Iatrogenic
Not yet classified

on which the shelf exam will test you: (1) Prophylactic Management (PPx), (2) Mechanism of Disease (MoD), (3) Diagnosis (Dx), and (4) Treatment/Management (Tx/Mgmt).

Benign Cysts and Neoplasms of the Ovary

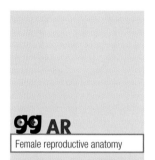

99 AR
Female reproductive anatomy

Adnexal masses, which are often not straightforward to manage and diagnose, are a commonly encountered entity in gynecology. They may be entirely asymptomatic and present incidentally, or may present with acute ovarian torsion or rupture, requiring surgical intervention. Physicians must thus determine the probability of the mass being malignant or the likelihood of it causing ovarian torsion to decide whether to manage the patient conservatively ("watch and wait") or with surgery.

There are a few situations involving adnexal masses that are considered medical emergencies: ovarian torsion, ruptured hemorrhagic ovarian cysts, and tubo-ovarian abscesses. The latter will be discussed more thoroughly in the chapter covering infections of the gynecologic tract.

The best initial technique for diagnosing and characterizing an adnexal mass or cyst is transvaginal ultrasound (TVUS), occasionally augmented by additional imaging with transabdominal ultrasound or cross-sectional imaging.

Functional (Physiologic) Ovarian Cyst

Buzz Words: Asymptomatic adnexal mass + anechoic + unilocular + simple, homogenous cyst

Clinical Presentation: A reproductive-aged woman who has no symptoms. The patient may have acute abdominal/pelvic pain if the cyst ruptures or if ovarian torsion has occurred.

Prophylaxis (PPx): N/A

Mechanism of Disease (MoD): A normal ovarian follicle fails to rupture during ovulation and continues to grow, stimulated by reproductive hormones. Functional ovarian cysts may become hemorrhagic due to bleeding within the cyst (Figs. 5.1 and 5.2).

99 AR
Ovarian neoplasms overview

Diagnostic Steps (Dx):

1. TVUS: The cyst is typically visualized as an anechoic (black) simple unilocular thin-walled cyst. These can become relatively large but are usually <10 cm (Fig. 5.3).

Treatment and Management Steps (Tx/Mgmt):

1. **Adnexal mass < 5 cm** → likely a functional ovarian cyst and may be observed. Repeat TVUS 6–8 weeks later typically reveals a smaller or resolved cyst. A physiologic follicular cyst should regress after the next menstrual period.

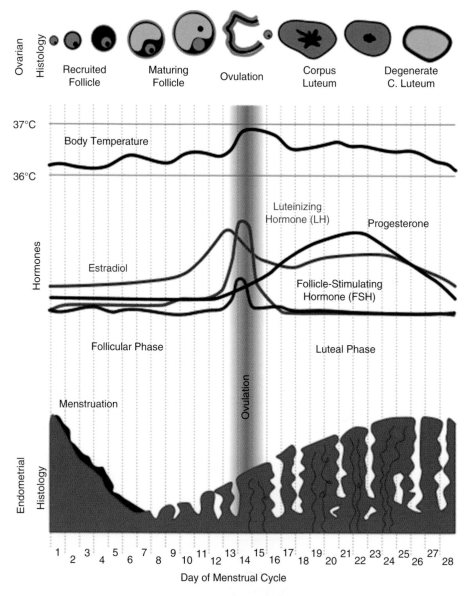

FIG. 5.1 The ovarian follicular cycle. (From Wiki Commons, Speck-Made, 2/25/2011 https://commons.wikimedia.org/wiki/File:MenstrualCycle_en.svg.)

2. Adnexal mass >10 cm → greater probability of being a tumor and more likely to cause ovarian torsion and therefore should be excised for pathologic evaluation.
3. Adnexal mass between 5 and 10 cm → acceptable to either observe with repeat imaging or surgically excise.

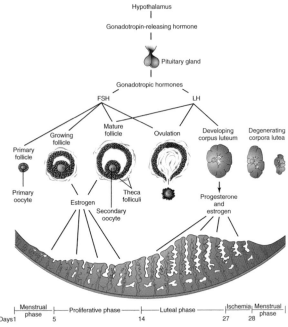

FIG. 5.2 Hormonal regulation of the ovarian follicular cycle. *FSH*, Follicle-stimulating hormone; LH, luteinizing hormone. (Modified [by Esther Baranov] from 2 images Elsevier Clinical Key: Figure 2.7. First week of human development. Moore KL, Torchia MG: *The developing human*, Chapter 2, pp 11–37.e1; and Figure 55.2. The female reproductive system. Mesiano S, Jones EE: *Medical physiology*, Chapter 55, pp 1108–1128.e1.)

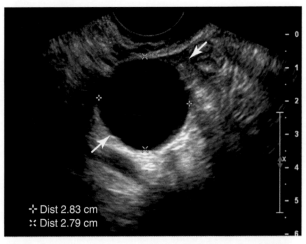

FIG. 5.3 Transvaginal ultrasound image of a simple cyst, exhibiting a thin-walled anechoic unilocular cyst. (From Elsevier Clinical Key: Figure 24.8. Adnexa. Hertzberg BS, Middleton WD: *Ultrasound: the requisites*, Chapter 24, pp 565–599.)

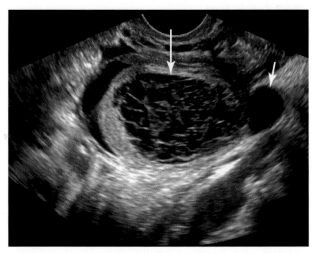

FIG. 5.4 Transvaginal ultrasound image of a hemorrhagic cyst, exhibiting the classic reticular "fishnet" pattern of internal echoes seen with organized hemorrhagic cysts. (From Elsevier Clinical Key: Figure 24.20. Adnexa. Hertzberg BS, Middleton WD: *Ultrasound: the requisites*, Chapter 24, pp 565–599.)

4. Cysts that are symptomatic, enlarging, persistent, or contain thick septations, papillary vegetations, or solid components are suspicious for malignancy and should be excised immediately.

Luteal Cyst

Buzz Words: Cystic adnexal mass + **"fishnet" reticular pattern on TVUS** + hemorrhagic cyst + early pregnancy

Clinical Presentation: A reproductive-aged woman who has no symptoms. The patient may have acute abdominal/pelvic pain if the cyst ruptures or if ovarian torsion has occurred.

PPx: N/A

MoD: A normal corpus luteum that fails to involute and continues to grow, stimulated by reproductive hormones. Corpus luteal cysts may become hemorrhagic.

Dx:
1. TVUS (Fig. 5.4):
   - Simple cyst (anechoic, uniloculated, smooth-walled)
   - Complex cyst (multiloculated, thick-walled, contain internal debris, a fluid level indicating recent hemorrhage)
   - Classic "fishnet" reticular pattern = hemorrhagic cyst

Tx/Mgmt:
1. Same as for functional ovarian cysts (see above)

QUICK TIP

High human chorionic gonadotropin (hCG) levels can be the
result of gestational trophoblastic
disease, multiple gestation, or
ovarian hyperstimulation due to
induction of ovulation for infertility
treatment.

Theca Lutein Cyst

Buzz Words: Bilateral, multilocular cystic adnexal masses +
"hyperreactio luteinalis" + **maternal** virilization + molar
pregnancy + fertility treatment

Clinical Presentation: A reproductive-aged woman who is
often asymptomatic, but may present with hyperemesis gravidarum, preeclampsia, thyroid dysfunction, or
features of maternal virilization. The patient may have
a history of fertility treatment, gestational trophoblastic disease (hydatidiform mole), multiple gestations, or
pregnancy with fetal hydrops.

PPx: N/A

MoD: Physiological follicular cysts that are luteinized by
overstimulation by extremely high levels of hCG during an abnormal pregnancy (or fertility treatments) or
heightened sensitivity to hCG during a normal pregnancy.

Dx:

1. TVUS → multiloculated cystic adnexal masses, often
   bilateral (Fig. 5.5)

Tx/Mgmt:

1. Treat the underlying etiology of high hCG.
2. Theca lutein cysts will resolve slowly (weeks to
   months) after removing the source of excessive hCG.

Endometrioma

Buzz Words: Chocolate cyst + "ground-glass" on TVUS +
endometriosis

Clinical Presentation: A reproductive-aged woman presenting with pelvic pain, dysmenorrhea, dyspareunia
(symptoms of endometriosis), or acute abdominal/pel-
vic pain if cyst rupture or ovarian torsion has occurred
(Fig. 5.6).

PPx: N/A

MoD: A manifestation of endometriosis: Ectopic growth
of endometrial tissue in the ovary bleeds and forms
a hematoma in a cyst lined by endometrial tissue.
Endometriomas often form multiple adhesions to surrounding pelvic structures, causing pain and obstruction.

Dx:

1. TVUS → cystic mass with homogeneous internal
   echoes ("ground glass" appearance), small hyperechoic foci in the cyst wall, and no solid component
   (Fig. 5.7).
2. Final diagnosis is confirmed by histologic evaluation of
   the surgical specimen following laparoscopy.

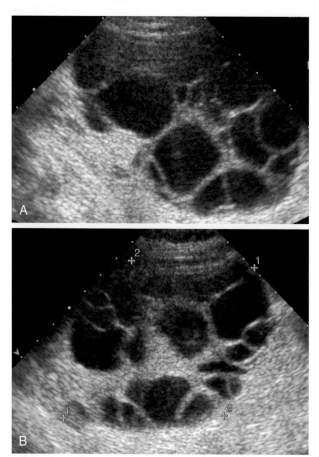

FIG. 5.5 Transvaginal ultrasound images of bilateral multiloculated simple cysts, consistent with theca lutein cysts. (From Elsevier Clinical Key: Figure T3.2. Theca lutein cyst. Benacerraf BR, Goldstein SR, Groszmann YS: *Gynecologic ultrasound: a problem-based approach*, pp 194–195.)

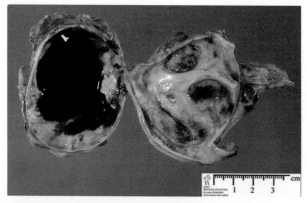

FIG. 5.6 Gross pathology image of a "chocolate-cyst" (endometrioma) cut open to reveal a fibrous capsule and chocolate-like cystic contents. (http://www.webpathology.com/image.asp?n=2&Case=524)

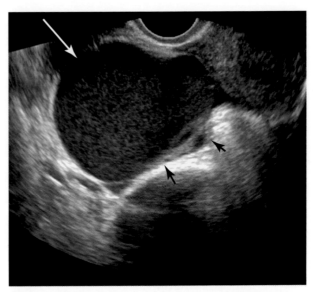

FIG. 5.7 Transvaginal ultrasound image of an endometrioma, displaying classic "ground glass" homogeneous internal echoes and hyperechoic foci *(black arrows)* in the cyst wall. (From Elsevier Clinical Key: Figure 24.22 [A]. Adnexa. Hertzberg BS, Middleton WD: *Ultrasound: the requisites*, Chapter 24, pp 565–599.)

Tx/Mgmt:

1. Same as for functional ovarian cysts (see above).
2. Symptomatic or enlarging endometriomas should be surgically excised (cystectomy), whereas small (<5 cm) or asymptomatic endometriomas should be observed.
3. Patients who undergo cystectomy should be prescribed oral contraceptives postoperatively as these have been shown to reduce recurrence of endometriomas.

Serous Cystadenoma

Buzz Words: Cystic adnexal mass + simple cyst (often)

Clinical Presentation: A reproductive-aged woman who has no symptoms. The patient may have acute abdominal/pelvic pain if the cyst ruptures or if ovarian torsion has occurred.

PPx: N/A

MoD: A benign cystic proliferation of ovarian surface epithelium that manifests as a fluid-filled cyst lined by a single layer of ciliated cells (recapitulates ciliated secretory epithelium of fallopian tubes).

Dx:

1. TVUS → larger (>5 cm) unilocular or multilocular simple cyst (anechoic, thin- and smooth-walled) with varying amounts of fibromatous stroma (Fig. 5.8).

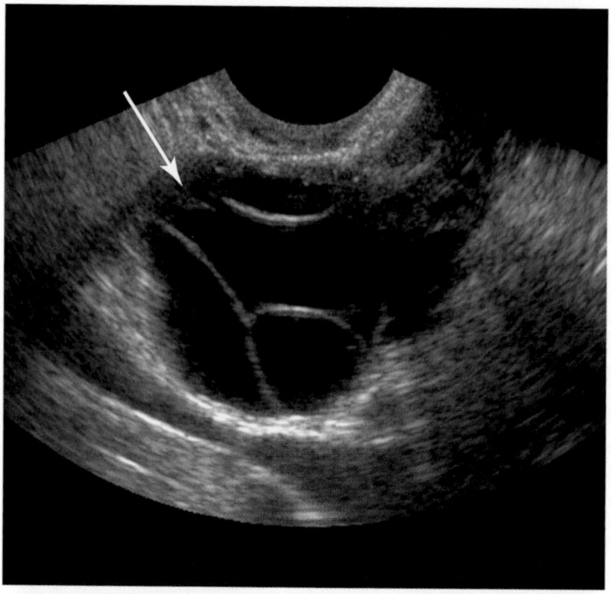

FIG. 5.8 Transvaginal ultrasound image of an ovarian serous cystadenoma, exhibiting an anechoic multiloculated cyst with thin septations. (From Elsevier Clinical Key: Figure 24.39 [A]. Adnexa. Hertzberg BS, Middleton WD: *Ultrasound: the requisites*, Chapter 24, pp 565–599.)

2. Final diagnosis is confirmed by histologic evaluation of the surgical specimen (Fig. 5.9).

Tx/Mgmt:

1. Same as for functional ovarian cysts (see above)—symptomatic or enlarging cystadenomas should be surgically excised.

Mucinous Cystadenoma

Buzz Words: Cystic adnexal mass + multiloculated

Clinical Presentation: A reproductive-aged woman, often with no symptoms, but may present with pressure, pain, bloating, or urinary symptoms if the cystadenomas grow large.

PPx: N/A

MoD: A benign cystic proliferation of ovarian surface epithelium that manifests as a fluid-filled cyst lined by a single layer of endocervical-like or intestinal-type epithelium (columnar cells containing apical intracytoplasmic mucin) and containing some amount of stroma.

Dx:

1. TVUS → very large, smooth-walled multiloculated cyst with varying amounts of fibromatous stroma. Rarely bilateral (Fig. 5.10).

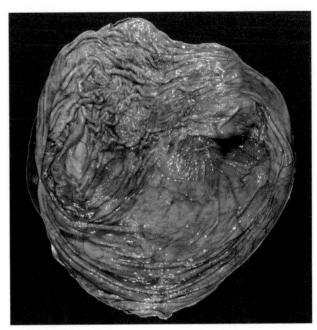

FIG. 5.9 Gross pathology image of a serous cystadenoma cut open to reveal a simple cyst with smooth thin walls. (Modified [by Esther Baranov] from Elsevier Clinical Key: Figure 39.10. Ovaries. Weidner N, Dabbs DJ, Peterson M: *Modern surgical pathology*, Chapter 39, pp 1356–1408.)

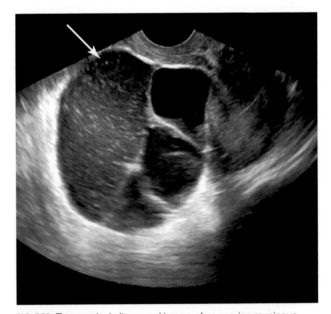

FIG. 5.10 Transvaginal ultrasound image of an ovarian mucinous cystadenoma, revealing a multilocular cystic mass containing areas of medium-level internal echoes *(white arrow)* that represent mucinous contents. (From Elsevier Clinical Key: Figure 24.39 [D]. Adnexa. Hertzberg BS, Middleton WD: *Ultrasound: the requisites*, Chapter 24, pp 565–599.)

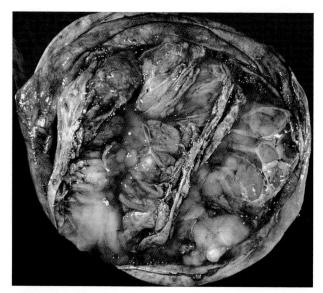

FIG. 5.11 Gross pathology image of a mucinous cystadenoma cut open to reveal a multiloculated cyst with smooth thin walls and septations. (Modified [by Esther Baranov] from Elsevier Clinical Key: Figure 10.5. The adnexal mass. McMeekin DS, Mannel RS, Di Saia PJ: *Clinical gynecologic oncology*, Chapter 10, pp 261–283.e4.)

2. Final diagnosis is confirmed by histologic evaluation of the surgical specimen.
3. *Note*: If mostly composed of fibromatous stroma, it is classified as mucinous adenofibroma or cystadenofibroma (Fig. 5.11).

Tx/Mgmt:
1. Same as for functional ovarian cysts (see above)— symptomatic or enlarging cystadenomas should be surgically excised.

Mature Cystic Teratoma ("Dermoid Cyst")

Buzz Words: "Dermoid cyst" + complex adnexal mass + bright linear echoes on TVUS + **cyst containing hair, bone, teeth, cartilage**

Clinical Presentation: The most common ovarian neoplasm (20%–40%). Patients are often reproductive-aged women with no symptoms. Patients may have acute abdominal/pelvic pain if the cyst ruptures or if ovarian torsion has occurred.

PPx: N/A

MoD: A benign cystic ovarian germ cell neoplasm arising from the three embryonic layers and containing a variety of mature tissues derived from these layers (hair, bone, teeth, cartilage, skin, etc.) caused by the proliferation of abnormal germ cells due to fusion of the

QUICK TIP

Rare forms of mature cystic teratoma include monodermal teratomas such as "struma ovarii"—a monodermal teratoma containing only or predominantly thyroid tissue and occasionally causing hyperthyroidism (though most often asymptomatic).

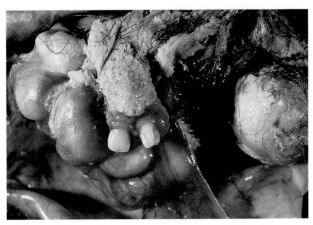

FIG. 5.12 Mature cystic teratoma cut open to reveal hair, teeth, sebaceous material, and other mature tissues filling the cystic cavity. (From Elsevier Clinical Key: Figure 19.290. Female reproductive system. Rosai J: *Rosai & Ackerman's surgical pathology*, 19, pp 1399–1657.)

ovum with the second polar body or due to failure of meiosis II.

Dx:

1. TVUS → cystic mass containing hyperechoic nodules with distal acoustic shadowing. May also appear uniformly hyperechoic or with bright linear echoes ("dermoid mesh") (Fig. 5.12).
2. Final diagnosis is confirmed by histologic evaluation of the surgical specimen (Fig. 5.13).

Tx/Mgmt:

1. **Cystectomy:** Recommended for definitive diagnosis and eliminating the possibility of ovarian torsion, cyst rupture, or malignant transformation.

Brenner Tumor (Transitional Cell Adenofibroma)

Buzz Words: Solid adnexal mass + transitional-type/urothelial epithelium

Clinical Presentation: Asymptomatic and often found incidentally during laparotomy for unrelated pelvic surgery.

PPx: N/A

MoD: Benign neoplasm of transitional-type (urothelial) epithelium that arose from ovarian surface epithelium via metaplasia.

Dx:

1. TVUS → unilateral, well-circumscribed, predominantly solid mass with scattered small cysts.
2. 25% are associated with a cystadenoma or mature dermoid cyst.
3. Final diagnosis is confirmed by histologic evaluation of the surgical specimen (Fig. 5.14).

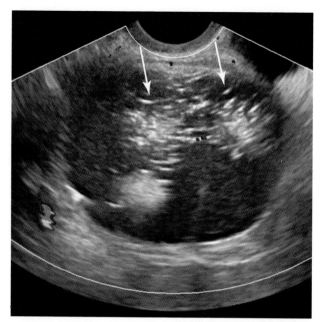

FIG. 5.13 Transvaginal ultrasound image of a mature cystic teratoma revealing a "dermoid mesh" of interlacing bright linear echoes *(white arrows)*, which correspond to hair strands within the cystic mass. (From Elsevier Clinical Key: Figure 24.36 [E]. Adnexa. Hertzberg BS, Middleton WD: *Ultrasound: the requisites*, Chapter 24, pp 565–599.)

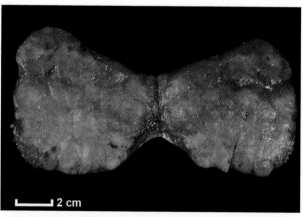

FIG. 5.14 Gross pathology image of a Brenner tumor cut open to reveal a well-circumscribed, lobulated, tan-yellow fibrous surface. (From Elsevier Clinical Key: Figure 11.36. Surface epithelial stromal tumors of the ovary. Longacre TA, Gilks CB: *Gynecologic pathology: a volume in the series: foundations in diagnostic pathology*, Chapter 11, pp 393–444.)

99 AR

Epithelial ovarian tumors

99 AR

Sex cord stromal ovarian tumors

Tx/Mgmt:

1. Salpingo-oophorectomy for conclusive diagnosis and to rule out a malignant component.

Malignant Neoplasms of the Ovary

In the United States, ovarian cancer is the second most prevalent cancer of the gynecologic tract and the most common cause of death from gynecologic malignancies. With only about 20% of ovarian carcinomas diagnosed as stage I, the majority present with metastatic disease at diagnosis, leading to poor overall prognosis and survival rates for ovarian cancer.

Ovarian cancers can be broken down by cell of origin into three main varieties: **epithelial ovarian carcinomas (EOCs),** which arise from the ovarian surface epithelium; **ovarian germ cell tumors (OGCTs),** which arise from primordial germ cells (PGCs); and **ovarian sex-cord stromal tumors (SCSTs),** which arise from ovarian sex-cord and stromal cells. The clear majority (95%) of ovarian carcinomas are epithelial in origin.

Aggressive surgery to remove all grossly visible disease is required for definitive diagnosis and cancer staging. A bilateral salpingo-oophorectomy (BSO), total abdominal hysterectomy (TAH), and lymph node dissection (pelvic and para-aortic) are standard for surgical staging of ovarian cancer. Resection of the omentum (omentectomy) is routinely performed to reduce tumor burden and decrease postoperative ascites accumulation and especially if omental caking (studding of the omentum with numerous small metastases) is noted. In addition to an omentectomy, the surgeon may perform an appendectomy, splenectomy, partial hepatectomy, diaphragmatic resection, and/or bowel resection. These extensive surgeries can be highly morbid and delay chemotherapy; however, overall survival has been shown to increase significantly when intraparenchymal metastases (such as those to spleen, liver, and bowel) are excised via aggressive surgery. In fact, overall survival is inversely correlated with the amount of residual tumor that remains after the initial surgery. Therefore, it is crucial for the surgeon to remove as much of the tumor and local metastases as possible during the initial surgery.

Complete cytoreduction is achieved when no grossly visible disease remains in the abdominal cavity after surgery. Optimal cytoreduction is achieved when all visible residual disease is less than 1 cm in maximum diameter. Patients with more complete cytoreductions survive significantly longer.

Appropriate staging also requires collection of ascites fluid if present or peritoneal washings if preoperative

TABLE 5.1 International Federation of Gynecology and Obstetrics 2014 Staging of Ovarian, Fallopian Tubal, and Peritoneal Cancer[a]

Stage	Extent of Disease	5-Year Survival
I	Tumor limited to ovaries/fallopian tubes	~85%–90%
IA	One ovary or fallopian tube involved	
IB	Both ovaries or fallopian tubes involved	
IC	IA or IB with surgical capsule rupture (IC1), preoperative capsule rupture or ovarian surface involvement (IC2), or malignant cells in ascites/peritoneal washings (IC3)	
II	Tumor limited to pelvis (below pelvic brim)	~65%–70%
IIA	Extension to uterus and/or fallopian tubes	
IIB	Extension to other pelvic tissues, including dense adhesions with histologically proven tumor cells	
III	Tumor limited to abdominal peritoneum (above pelvic brim)	~35%–45%
IIIA	Positive retroperitoneal lymph nodes (IIIA1) ± microscopic peritoneal metastases (IIIA2)	
IIIB	Macroscopic peritoneal metastases (up to 2 cm) ± positive retroperitoneal lymph nodes	
IIIC	Macroscopic peritoneal metastases (>2 cm) including to liver/spleen capsule ± positive retroperitoneal lymph nodes	
IV	Distant metastases	~20%
IVA	Pleural effusion with malignant cytology	
IVB	Parenchymal metastases to intra- or extra-abdominal organs (including inguinal or extra-abdominal lymph nodes)	

[a]Details such as subdivisions of stage IC and IIIA are stated here for completion, but are low-yield for shelf examinations.

or intraoperative capsule rupture are suspected. These should be collected as soon as the abdomen is open and sent for cytology. Pleural effusions should also be drained and sent for cytology, as pleural effusions positive for malignant cells upstage the patient to stage IVA (Table 5.1). Additionally, biopsies of diaphragmatic implants or other suspected metastases are taken for complete staging purposes.

Epithelial Ovarian Carcinoma

Types:
- Serous adenocarcinoma (high- or low-grade):
  - Composed of fallopian tubal-type epithelium, approximately 60% bilateral
  - Most common subtype (75%)
  - High-grade: *BRCA1/BRCA2* (germline or somatic) and *TP53* mutations
  - Low-grade: *K-RAS* and *BRAF* mutations
- Mucinous adenocarcinoma:
  - Composed of mucinous endocervical-like or intestinal-type epithelium, most often unilateral

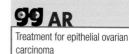

Treatment for epithelial ovarian carcinoma

- <10% of all EOCs
- *K-RAS* mutations
- NO association with *BRCA1/BRCA2* mutations
- Endometrioid adenocarcinoma:
  - Germline mutations in DNA mismatch repair genes (hereditary nonpolyposis colorectal cancer [HNPCC]), microsatellite instability, or *PTEN* and *β-catenin* somatic mutations
- Clear-cell adenocarcinoma
- Transitional-cell adenocarcinoma

Buzz Words: Complex cystic mass + postmenopausal woman + younger woman with *BRCA* germline mutation + weight loss + early satiety + pelvic pressure/pain + malignant pleural effusion + ascites

Clinical Presentation: A postmenopausal female (50s–70s) or adult female (30s–40s) with hereditary ovarian cancer syndromes (e.g., *BRCA* mutations) presents with weight loss, vague pressure and pain, bloating, and early satiety. Some may present acutely with bowel obstruction due to compression of the bowel by an enlarging ovarian mass or shortness of breath due to malignant pleural effusion.

Risk Factors:
- Age: Incidence of epithelial ovarian cancer increases with age.
- Hereditary ovarian cancer syndromes: *BRCA1/BRCA2* gene mutation, HNPCC
- Infertility or nulliparity
- PCOS
- Early menarche (before 12) or late menopause (after 52)
- Cigarette smoking (increases risk of mucinous subtype)
- Endometriosis (increases risk of endometrioid, clear-cell, and low-grade serous subtypes)
- First-degree relatives with ovarian cancer

PPx: Oral contraceptive use, breast feeding, tubal ligation, or salpingo-oophorectomy. Pregnancy and multiparity are associated with a reduced risk of ovarian cancer, which is believed to be due to fewer years a woman spends ovulating.

MoD: (Fig. 5.15)

1. **High-grade carcinomas** are thought to arise from cortical inclusion cysts (Fig. 5.16) in the ovaries or from precursor lesions of the fimbriated end of the fallopian tubes (known as serous tubal intraepithelial carcinoma [STIC] lesions). High-grade lesions evolve rapidly and have a high cellular proliferation rate, mutations in *BRCA* genes and *TP53*, and a significantly lower 5-year survival rate than their low-grade counterparts (Fig. 5.17).

QUICK TIP

STIC lesions were discovered in surgical specimens from women undergoing risk-reducing bilateral salpingo-oophorectomy (rrBSO) for known germline *BRCA1* or *BRCA2* mutations.

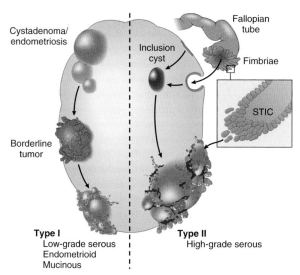

FIG. 5.15 Proposed pathogenesis of different types of ovarian carcinoma. Note that one pathway for high-grade serous carcinoma involves serous tubal intraepithelial carcinoma (STIC) cells from the fimbriated end of the fallopian tube implanting on the surface of the ovary. (From Elsevier Clinical Key: Figure 22.30. The female genital tract. Ellenson LH, Pirog EC: *Robbins and Cotran pathologic basis of disease*, Chapter 22, pp 991–1042.)

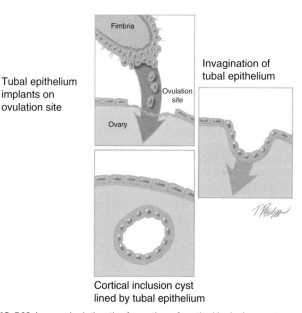

FIG. 5.16 Image depicting the formation of cortical inclusion cysts lined by fallopian tubal epithelium. (From Elsevier Clinical Key: Figure 7. Kurman RJ, Shih IM: Molecular pathogenesis and extraovarian origin of epithelial ovarian cancer—shifting the paradigm. *Hum Pathol* 42[7]:918–931, 2011.)

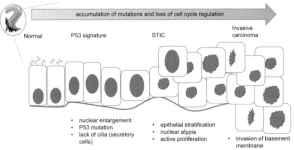

FIG. 5.17 Oncogenesis of high-grade serous ovarian carcinoma. *STIC*, Serous tubal intraepithelial carcinoma. (From Elsevier Clinical Key: Reade CJ, McVey RM, Tone AA, Finlayson SJ, McAlpine JN, Fung-Kee-Fung M, Ferguson SE: The fallopian tube as the origin of high grade serous ovarian cancer: review of a paradigm shift. *J Obstet Gynaecol Can* 36[2]:133–140, 2014, Copyright © 2014 Society of Obstetricians and Gynaecologists of Canada.)

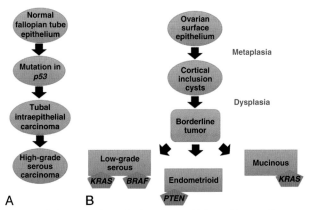

FIG. 5.18 Schematic of genetic alterations in high- and low-grade serous ovarian carcinoma. (From Elsevier Clinical Key: Figure 1. Epigenetic pathways offer targets for ovarian cancer treatment. Article in Press: Corrected Proof. Gyparaki MT, Papavassiliou AG: *Clinical ovarian and other gynecologic cancer*, Copyright © 2015 The Authors.)

2. **Low-grade carcinomas** and other subtypes are believed to arise from repetitive ovulation (secondary to nulliparity, PCOS, early menarche, late menopause), causing oxidative damage to the surface epithelium and cortical inclusion cysts, which eventually lead to malignant transformation and carcinoma. Low-grade lesions grow slowly, are thought to progress through benign and borderline lesions, and have a low cellular proliferation rate with mutations in *BRAF* and *K-RAS* rather than *BRCA* or *TP53* (Fig. 5.18).

Dx:

1. Elevated CA-125 in 80% of cases
2. TVUS → large, complex, cystic mass with solid components, septations, and thick irregular walls

3. Follow-up studies with magnetic resonance imaging (MRI) or computed tomography (CT) may reveal ascites, pleural effusions, or peritoneal implants.
4. Final diagnosis is confirmed by histologic evaluation of surgical specimen.

Tx/Mgmt:

1. Surgery for staging and treatment typically involves a BSO and TAH, and may include a lymph node dissection, omentectomy, appendectomy, splenectomy, partial hepatectomy, diaphragmatic resection, and/or bowel resection.
2. Rupturing the cystic mass and spilling malignant contents into the peritoneal cavity up-stages the patient, and thus aspiration or biopsy prior to surgical removal are not performed.
3. High-grade serous carcinoma is more likely to respond to chemotherapy (platinum-sensitive) than low-grade serous carcinoma (often platinum-insensitive), but low-grade carcinoma has a more indolent course and better prognosis.

Ovarian Germ Cell Tumors

Definition: Neoplasms derived from PGCs, accounting for the majority of ovarian tumors occurring in the first two decades of life:

- **Teratoma**—mature cystic teratoma (benign, most common primary ovarian neoplasm, rarely can undergo malignant degeneration), immature teratoma (malignant).

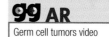
Germ cell tumors video

- **Dysgerminoma**—comprised of immature cells that resemble PGCs, morphologically resembling seminomas (in males) and extragonadal germinomas. Dysgerminomas make up 50% of malignant germ cell tumors but only 1% of all ovarian cancers.
- **Yolk sac tumor**—comprised of PGCs that differentiate toward yolk sac and primitive placenta forms, or embryonic forms. Yolk sac tumors are the second most common germ cell tumors.
- **Mixed germ cell tumor**—combination of germ cell tumors or gonadoblastoma (mixed germ cell-sex cord-stromal tumor typically seen with disorders of sexual development such as complete androgen insensitivity or gonadal dysgenesis).

Buzz Words: Rapidly growing mass + immature germ cells + young/teenage girl + ovarian torsion + vaginal bleeding (Fig. 5.19)

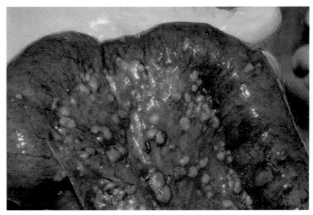

FIG. 5.19 Intraoperative image of multiple metastatic foci of ovarian carcinoma on the small bowel mesentery (peritoneal carcinomatosis). These should be removed for optimal cytoreduction and sent for pathology, especially if they are greater than 1 cm in diameter. (From Elsevier Clinical Key: Figure 39.1. Ovarian, fallopian tube, and peritoneal cancer. Berek JS: *Hacker & Moore's essentials of obstetrics and gynecology*, Chapter 39, pp 440–448.)

Clinical Presentation:
- Dysgerminoma:
  - Age: 20s–30s, up to 20% of dysgerminomas are diagnosed during pregnancy!
  - Chief Complaint: Pain/pressure due to rapidly growing pelvic mass, abdominal enlargement, can present acutely with ovarian torsion or rupture, or may have irregular vaginal bleeding or pregnancy-like symptoms due to elevated serum β-hCG.
- Yolk sac tumors:
  - Age: 0–20
  - Chief Complaint: Pain/pressure due to rapidly growing pelvic mass, abdominal enlargement, can present acutely with ovarian torsion or rupture.

PPx: None

MoD: May arise from primordial germ cells, which migrate from the yolk sac to the primitive gonadal ridge during embryogenesis. These precursor cells give rise to histologically similar tumors in males and females (e.g., seminoma and dysgerminoma).

Dx:
1. Dysgerminomas:
   - Elevated serum levels of β-hCG, lactate dehydrogenase (LDH), and placental alkaline phosphatase (PLAP)
   - TVUS → solid ovarian mass with fibrovascular septations separating multiple nodules; may see calcifications in a speckled pattern

- Final diagnosis is confirmed by histologic evaluation of surgical specimen.
2. Yolk sac tumors:
   - Elevated serum levels of alpha-fetoprotein (AFP) and CA-125
   - TVUS → complex, cystic mass
   - Final diagnosis is confirmed by histologic evaluation of surgical specimen.

Tx/Mgmt:
1. Due to the less aggressive nature of these tumors (compared to epithelial ovarian cancer), more conservative fertility-sparing surgery is acceptable for stage I tumors.
2. Those with extraovarian disease require salpingo-oophorectomy and optimal debulking (cytoreduction), which can include TAH and omentectomy, followed by multiagent chemotherapy. BEP (bleomycin, etoposide, and cisplatin) is the most commonly used chemotherapy regimen.
3. Surveillance for recurrence of dysgerminomas includes monitoring of LDH, PLAP and β-HCG, while for yolk sack tumors AFP serum levels are monitored.

Ovarian Sex-Cord Stromal Tumor

Definition: Heterogeneous group of rare benign or malignant neoplasms derived from stems cells of ovarian or testicular stroma, sub-classified by the WHO as follows:
- **Granulosa stromal cell tumors (70% of SCSTs)**—e.g., thecoma, fibroma, granulosa cell tumors
- **Sertoli stromal cell tumors**—e.g., Sertoli-Leydig cell tumors, Sertoli cell tumors
- **Mixed or unclassified SCSTs**—e.g., gynandroblastoma (exceedingly rare)
- **Steroid cell tumors**—e.g., stromal luteoma

Buzz Words:
- **Granulosa cell tumors**: PMB in postmenopausal woman or precocious puberty in prepubertal girl + abdominal enlargement + estrogen elevated
- **Sertoli-Leydig cell tumors**: Reproductive-aged woman + virilization (acne, alopecia, voice deepening, hirsutism) + abdominal enlargement

Clinical Presentation:
- **Granulosa cell tumors:**
   - Age: wide age range
   - Chief Complaint: Abdominal enlargement, pressure and pain; can present with precocious puberty, PMB, or menorrhagia due to production of excess estrogen by tumor.

- PMH (past medical history): Associated with EC in 15%
- Sertoli-Leydig cell tumors:
  1. Age: 15–35, younger reproductive-aged women
  2. Chief Complaint: Abdominal enlargement, pressure, and pain; may present with signs of virilization (acne, menstrual irregularity, alopecia, voice deepening, hirsutism, clitoral enlargement) due to production of excess androgens by tumor.

PPx: N/A

MoD: Arise from precursor cells of gonadal primitive sex-cords or stroma, which can differentiate toward male or female hormone-producing sex-cord cells (granulosa, theca, Sertoli, and Leydig cells) or stromal cells (fibroblasts), creating a heterogeneous group of rare neoplasms.

Dx:
1. Granulosa cell tumors:
   - TVUS → appear as large echogenic multilocular cystic or solid adnexal masses, often with thickened endometrium.
   - High inhibin levels in a postmenopausal woman or in a premenopausal woman with amenorrhea are suggestive.
   - Final diagnosis is confirmed by histologic evaluation of surgical specimen.
2. Sertoli-Leydig cell tumors:
   - TVUS → large solid adnexal masses
   - High serum androgen levels (testosterone, dehydro-epiandrosterone [DHEA])
   - Final diagnosis is confirmed by histologic evaluation of surgical specimen.

Tx/Mgmt:
1. Unilateral salpingo-oophorectomy is acceptable for Stage Ia tumors.
2. TAH/BSO and platinum-based chemotherapy is used for poorly differentiated or higher-stage tumors or women who have completed childbearing.
3. Serum inhibin levels can be used to monitor for tumor recurrence in patients with granulosa cell tumors and serum testosterone levels can be used to monitor patients with Sertoli-Leydig tumors.

Benign Neoplasms of the Uterus

Endometrial Polyp

Definition: Proliferation of endometrial tissue that projects into the uterine cavity as a pedunculated polyp or sessile (flat, broad-based) polyp.

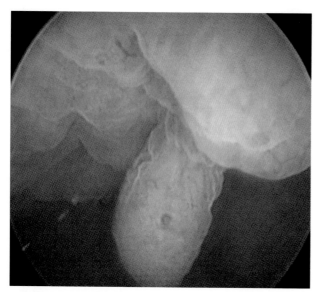

FIG. 5.20 Visualization of an endometrial polyp on hysteroscopy. (Modified [by Esther Baranov] from Elsevier Clinical Key: FIG. 5. Di Spiezio Sardo A, Calagna G, Guida M, Perino A, Nappi C: Hysteroscopy and treatment of uterine polyps. *Best Pract Res Clin Obstet Gynaecol* 29[7]:908–919, 2015.)

Buzz Words: Intermenstrual bleeding + postcoital spotting

Clinical Presentation: Most in women >40 who present with intermenstrual, postcoital, bleeding or spotting.

PPx: N/A

MoD: Proliferation of endometrial tissue with irregular gland architecture and dense fibrotic stroma.

Dx:

1. TVUS → polypoid or sessile mass visualized in endometrial cavity of uterus.
2. Final diagnosis is confirmed by histologic evaluation of surgical specimen. See Fig. 5.20.

Tx/Mgmt:

1. Visualization and removal (polypectomy/dilatation and curettage) so as not to mask other AUB.
2. Less than 5% are associated with malignancy.

Leiomyomata Uteri ("Fibroids," Uterine Leiomyomas)

Definition: Benign neoplasms of uterine smooth muscle with various locations in the uterus—submucosal, intramural, subserosal, or cervical. Leiomyomas are the most common pelvic tumors in women, with a slightly higher incidence in black women.

Buzz Words: AUB + dysmenorrhea + infertility + irregularly enlarged uterus

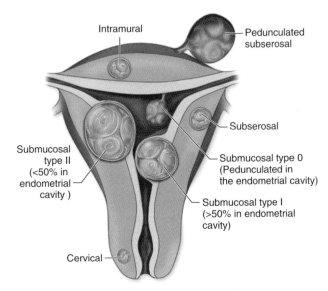

FIG. 5.21 Possible anatomic locations of uterine leiomyomas (fibroids). (Figure modified [by Esther Baranov] from Elsevier Clinical Key: Figure 15.1. Uterine leiomyomas. Brown DL: *Gynecologic imaging: expert radiology series*, Chapter 15, pp 237–250.)

Clinical Presentation: Reproductive-aged women (symptoms fade after menopause and leiomyomas shrink as hormone levels decline) who have heavy and/or prolonged vaginal bleeding, dysmenorrhea, pelvic pain or pressure, urinary frequency (compression of bladder), or constipation (compression of rectum). The patient may also have infertility or multiple spontaneous abortions (due to submucosal leiomyomas distorting the endometrial cavity) and anemia (secondary to heavy bleeding) (Fig. 5.21).

PPx: Prophylactic treatment of fibroids is not recommended.

MoD: Proliferation of smooth muscle cells of uterine myometrium

Dx:
1. Bimanual pelvic exam reveals large, irregularly shaped, but mobile uterus
2. TVUS → hypoechoic or heterogeneous mass. See Fig. 5.22.
3. Saline-infusion sonography (SIS) can better characterize intracavitary and submucosal fibroids than TVUS alone.
4. MRI, best modality for visualizing multiple leiomyomas in greatly enlarged uteri, is reserved for surgical planning.
5. Final diagnosis is confirmed by histologic evaluation of surgical specimen. See Fig. 5.23.

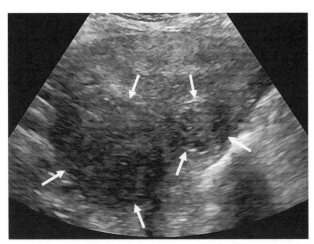

FIG. 5.22 Transvaginal ultrasound image of a uterus with two leiomyomas *(white arrows)*, visualized as well-circumscribed hypoechoic masses. (From Elsevier Clinical Key: Figure 1. Zampolin RL, Shi A: Radiologic evaluation of mesenchymal tumors of the female genital tract. *Surg Pathol Clin* 2[4]:581–602, 2009.)

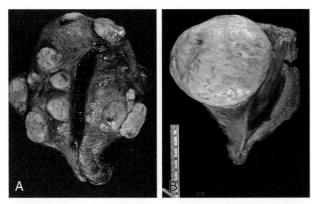

FIG. 5.23 Gross pathology images of uterine leiomyomas ("fibroids"). Note that one specimen has multiple smaller fibroids (A), whereas the other specimen has one large fibroid (B). Both can cause bulk symptoms and infertility due to their enlargement of the uterus and distortion of the uterine cavity, respectively. (Modified [by Esther Baranov] from 2 images Elsevier Clinical Key: Figures 19.167 and 19.168. Female reproductive system. Rosai J: *Rosai & Ackerman's surgical pathology*, 19, pp 1399–1657.)

Tx/Mgmt:
1. There are a variety of treatment modalities with the primary goal of eliminating symptoms and improving fertility:
   - **Expectant management** or "watchful waiting"— suitable for patients with asymptomatic or mildly symptomatic fibroids.
   - **Medical management** with oral contraceptives or levonorgestrel-releasing intrauterine device

(IUD)—suitable for patients who wish to try the least invasive option first.

- **Gonadotropin-releasing hormone (GnRH) agonists**—most effective medical treatment for fibroids; however, there is rapid regrowth of uterine size and menses following cessation of treatment. GnRH agonists cause a hypogonadotropic state (resembling menopause), causing a dramatic reduction in uterine fibroid size and amenorrhea within months. Long-term treatment is limited by osteoporosis and other symptoms caused by a hypoestrogenic state (hot flashes, mood disturbances, vaginal dryness). Due to these side effects, GnRH agonists are often used solely for preoperative reduction in uterine size.
- **Myomectomy** (hysteroscopic or laparoscopic/robotic depending on fibroid location)—surgical excision of fibroids—suitable for patients who wish to preserve fertility and/or have submucosal fibroids amenable to hysteroscopic myomectomy; however, fibroids often recur.
- **Hysterectomy**—surgical removal of uterus—performed in patients with multiple large fibroids, recurrence of symptoms after myomectomy, and no desire for future childbearing.
- **Uterine artery embolization**—for patients who no longer desire future childbearing but do not want to undergo surgery or wish to keep their uterus.
- **Note:** Patients with large fibroid(s) obstructing the fetus' ability to exit the vagina will require a C-section.

Malignant and Premalignant Neoplasms of the Uterus

Endometrial Hyperplasia

Definition: Proliferation of endometrial glands with irregular architecture resulting from chronic estrogen stimulation unopposed by progesterone:

- **Simple hyperplasia:** Mildly crowded, dilated cystic endometrial glands
- **Complex hyperplasia:** Crowded, disorganized endometrial glands
- **Nuclear atypia:** Nuclear enlargement (strongest prognostic factor for progression to endometrial carcinoma)

Buzz Words: PMB + unopposed estrogen + obesity + nulliparous, irregular menses + PCOS + thickened endometrial stripe

Clinical Presentation: A perimenopausal patient presents with heavy menses and intermenstrual bleeding.

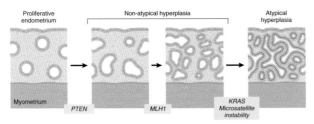

FIG. 5.24 Genetic mutations associated with atypical endometrial hyperplasia. (Modified [by Esther Baranov] from Elsevier Clinical Key: Figure 22.24. The female genital tract. Ellenson LH, Pirog EC: *Robbins and Cotran pathologic basis of disease*, Chapter 22, pp. 991–1042.)

- Risk factors for endometrial hyperplasia and cancer relate to unopposed estrogen:
  - Unopposed estrogen replacement therapy
  - Tamoxifen
  - Obesity (aromatization of androgens to estrogen in peripheral fat)
  - Diabetes
  - Chronic anovulatory cycles (irregular menses, PCOS)
  - Early menarche (before 12)
  - Late menopause (after 55)
  - Nulliparity
  - Older age
  - Family history of endometrial, breast, ovarian, or colon cancer
  - Lynch syndrome (HNPCC) or Cowden syndrome
  - Estrogen-secreting ovarian tumors (e.g., granulosa cell tumor)

PPx:
- Combined oral contraceptives (balance of estrogen and progesterone protective in individuals with anovulatory cycles or PCOS)
- Multiparity
- Weight loss (decreased synthesis of estrogen by peripheral fat)

MoD: Chronic exposure of the endometrium (lining of uterus) to endogenous or exogenous estrogen unopposed by the balancing effect of progesterone, stimulating endometrial glands to proliferate (endometrial hyperplasia) and accumulate genetic mutations (*PTEN*, *MLH1*, *KRAS*, microsatellite instability), causing nuclear atypia and potential for malignant transformation to EC. See Fig. 5.24.

Dx:
1. Pelvic exam and TVUS (r/o other etiologies for AUB are present, such as polyps or fibroids)

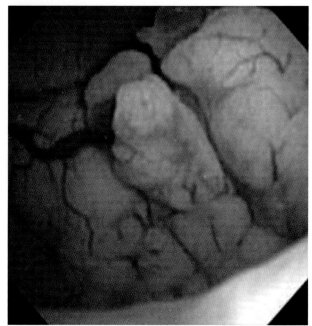

FIG. 5.25 Hysteroscopic view of endometrial hyperplasia. (From Elsevier Clinical Key: Figure 2. Oda K, Koga K, Hirata T, et al: Risk of endometrial cancer in patients with a preoperative diagnosis of atypical endometrial hyperplasia treated with total laparoscopic hysterectomy. *Gynecol Minim Invasive Therap* 5[2]:69–73, 2016.)

2. In postmenopausal women not on hormonal replacement therapy, measurement of endometrial stripe thickness on TVUS is an acceptable less invasive option for assessing women with suspicion for endometrial hyperplasia:
    • If the endometrial stripe thickness is <5 mm, it is acceptable to hold off on immediate endometrial sampling (biopsy or curettage) in these women.
    • If the endometrium is not adequately visualized on TVUS or the patient continues to experience persistent vaginal bleeding despite a stripe thickness of 5 mm or greater, endometrial biopsy must be performed.
3. Definitive diagnosis of endometrial hyperplasia is by histology on endometrial biopsy, endometrial curettage, or hysterectomy specimens (Fig. 5.25).

Tx/Mgmt:

1. Management of endometrial hyperplasia depends on the presence or absence of nuclear atypia.
    • **Hyperplasia without nuclear atypia**—low risk of progression to EC (1%–3%):
        • Progestin therapy to balance unopposed estrogen, reverse endometrial hyperplasia, and removal of the source of estrogen if possible

QUICK TIP

TVUS should NOT be used to determine endometrial stripe thickness in *pre*menopausal women because the thickness of the endometrium changes with the menstrual cycle and could be misleading. Premenopausal women with suspicion for endometrial hyperplasia or carcinoma must undergo immediate endometrial biopsy.

(discontinuation of hormonal therapy, weight loss, removal of estrogen-secreting tumor).
- Repeat endometrial biopsy in 3 months to assess response.
- **Hyperplasia with nuclear atypia**—high risk of progression to EC (10%–30%):
  - If the patient is not considering future pregnancy and has completed childbearing, hysterectomy is recommended.
  - If the patient is considering future pregnancy, progestin therapy is appropriate until childbearing is complete.
  - In postmenopausal women, hysterectomy with BSO is recommended due to the relatively high risk of EC in this age group and possibility of occult metastasis to the ovaries.
  - In a patient with many risk factors (obesity, diabetes, PCOS) or with persistent PMB, if endometrial sampling reveals no hyperplasia or carcinoma, the patient must still undergo hysteroscopy for direct visualization of the uterine cavity and guided biopsy. Hysteroscopy may reveal small endometrial lesions or polyps (which may also be malignant) that were missed on initial endometrial biopsy due to sampling error.

Simple hyperplasia w/o atypia → 1% (penny)	Complex hyperplasia w/o atypia → 3% (nickel)
Simple hyperplasia w/ atypia → 8% (dime)	Complex hyperplasia w/ atypia → 29% (quarter)

Endometrial Cancer

EC is the most common gynecologic cancer in developed countries. It has a relatively good prognosis compared to ovarian cancer because approximately 70% of patients are diagnosed as stage I cancer, with a 5-year survival of approximately 90%. The prognosis for EC is based on stage, histological grade, and subtype. EC, like ovarian cancer, is staged surgically by performing a TAH, BSO, omentectomy, and intraoperative pelvic and para-aortic lymph node assessment and sampling (see Table 5.2).

Definition: It can be broken down histologically into two distinct types:
- **Type I endometrial cancer**: Low-grade (FIGO grade 1 and 2) endometrioid histology, most common EC (75%–80%), less aggressive, presents early with AUB, estrogen receptor (ER) positive,

QUICK TIP

Progestin activates progesterone receptors in the endometrium of the uterus, causing decidualization of the stroma and subsequent thinning of the endometrium while also downregulating estrogen and progesterone receptors in the endometrium, thus decreasing hyperplasia of endometrial glands.

QUICK TIP

Remember! Endometrial ablation for vaginal bleeding in patients with endometrial hyperplasia is *contraindicated* because it would prevent future evaluation of the endometrium by endometrial biopsy and could mask the development of premalignant or malignant lesions.

QUICK TIP

Risk of progression to endometrial cancer in four categories of endometrial hyperplasia. Nuclear atypia increases the risk of malignant transformation more so than complexity of the gland architecture! The percentage risk of progression can be easily remembered and closely approximated with the mnemonic "penny, nickel, dime, quarter," which stands for 1%, 5%, 10%, 25%.

QUICK TIP

Atrophic endometritis or vaginitis (friable atrophic tissue of the endometrium or vagina due to low estrogen levels in menopause) is the *most common* cause of postmenopausal bleeding. However, **endometrial cancer must be ruled out in any woman with postmenopausal bleeding.**

TABLE 5.2 International Federation for Gynecology and Obstetrics 2009 Staging of Endometrial Cancer[a]

Stage	Extent of Disease	5-Year Survival
I	Tumor limited to uterus (corpus uteri)	~80%–90%
IA	Tumor limited to endometrium or invades less than half of myometrium	
IB	Tumor invades half of myometrium or more	
II	Tumor extension to cervical stroma only	~75%
III	Tumor extension to regional structures and lymph nodes	~35%–55%
IIIA	Uterine serosa, pelvic peritoneum, and/or adnexa involved (via direct extension or metastasis)	
IIIB	Vagina and/or parametria involved (via direct extension or metastasis)	
IIIC	Metastases to pelvic lymph nodes (IIIC1) and/or para-aortic lymph nodes (IIIC2)	
IV	Tumor invasion of bladder/bowel or distant metastases	~20%–25%
IVA	Invasion of bladder and/or bowel mucosa	
IVB	Distant metastases to intra- or extra-abdominal organs (including inguinal lymph nodes)	

[a]Details such as subdivisions of stage IIIC are stated here for completion, but are ultimately low-yield in terms of shelf examinations.

postmenopausal women with classic risk factors or premenopausal women with chronic anovulation, PCOS, and/or obesity.

- **Type II endometrial cancer:** Serous, clear cell, mixed cell, or undifferentiated histology, or high-grade (FIGO 3) endometrioid histology, aggressive with poor prognosis, ER negative, thin patients, late menopausal patients, or patients without classic risk factors.

Buzz Words: PMB + unopposed estrogen + obesity + nulliparous, irregular menses + PCOS + thickened endometrial stripe

Clinical Presentation: A 55-year-old postmenopausal woman presents with vaginal bleeding.

- Risk factors:
  - Type I endometrial cancer has the same set of risk factors as for endometrial hyperplasia (see above).
  - Type II endometrial cancers are not associated with these classic risk factors, are not stimulated by estrogen (don't express estrogen or progesterone receptors), and typically arise in atrophic endometrium of older women.
  - Malignant mixed müllerian tumors (MMMTs); carcinosarcomas are associated with prior pelvic radiation.

PPx: Same as for endometrial hyperplasia (see above).

MoD:

- Type I endometrial cancer has the same mechanism of disease as its precursor lesion, endometrial

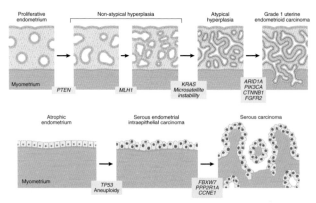

FIG. 5.26 Genetic mutations associated with endometrial cancer. *CTNNB1*, gene for β-catenin; *CCNE1*, gene for cyclin E1; *MLH1*, mismatch repair gene. (From Elsevier Clinical Key: Figure 22.24. The female genital tract. Ellenson LH, Pirog EC: *Robbins and Cotran pathologic basis of disease*, Chapter 22, pp 991–1042.)

hyperplasia (see above). There are multiple known genetic mutations that are believed to contribute to malignant transformation, including *PTEN, KRAS, MLH1* (leading to microsatellite instability), *PIK3CA*, and *β-catenin (CTNNB1)*. *PTEN* inactivation is thought to occur early on in carcinogenesis and can be seen in atypical endometrial hyperplasia. *MLH1*, one of the mismatch repair proteins, can be inactivated by DNA hypermethylation or as a germline mutation in patients with Lynch syndrome.

- Type II endometrial cancers are characterized by *TP53* mutations (Fig. 5.26).
- MMMTs are thought to arise from high-grade carcinomas with epithelial-to-mesenchymal transformation causing the sarcomatous component of the carcinosarcoma.
- Patients with Lynch syndrome (HNPCC) or Cowden syndrome have a hereditary predisposition for EC, with a lifetime risk of developing EC of approximately 60% and 10%, respectively:
  - **Lynch syndrome** (HNPCC) —germline mutations in mismatch repair proteins (*MLH1, MSH2, MSH6, PMS2*) predisposing to all histologic subtypes of EC, as well as colon and ovarian cancer.
  - **Cowden syndrome**—autosomal dominant germline mutation in *PTEN* predisposing to EC.

Dx:

1. Evaluation for EC is the same as for endometrial hyperplasia.
2. Final diagnosis is confirmed by histologic evaluation of the surgical specimen (Fig. 5.27).

QUICK TIP

Note that mutations in *PTEN* and *β-catenin* as well as microsatellite instability are implicated in carcinogenesis of endometrioid adenocarcinoma of the ovary.

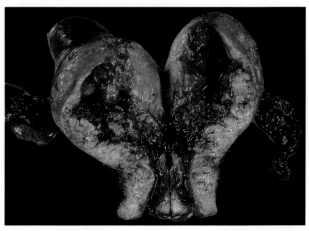

FIG. 5.27 Gross pathology image of a uterus with endometrial cancer. Note how the tumor infiltrates deeply into the myometrium and fills the endometrial cavity. (Modified [by Esther Baranov] from Elsevier Clinical Key. Figure. 19.136. Female reproductive system. Rosai J: *Rosai & Ackerman's surgical pathology*, 19, pp 1399–1657.)

Tx/Mgmt:

1. EC is staged *surgically* by performing a TAH, BSO, and intraoperative lymph node sampling.
2. Women with a family history suggestive of a hereditary cancer syndrome should undergo genetic testing for Lynch or Cowden syndrome.
3. Women with stage IA, FIGO grade 1 endometrial carcinoma who desire future childbearing are candidates for progestin therapy (and deferral of TAH-BSO until after childbearing) if a thorough initial medical evaluation reveals no evidence of high-stage or high-grade disease.

Hydatidiform Mole (Benign Gestational Trophoblastic Disease)

Definition: A product of aberrant fertilization of an ovum by 1 or 2 sperm that forms an abnormal placenta with cytogenetic abnormalities.

Buzz Words: Villous edema + molar pregnancy + vesicular bloody mass + "snowstorm" appearance on ultrasound (Fig. 5.28)

Clinical Presentation:

- Extremes of maternal age (<15 and >40)
- Complete moles may present with spontaneous abortion (vaginal bleeding and passage of vesicular mass), early preeclampsia (before 20 weeks), multiple theca lutein cysts causing ovarian enlargement, hyperemesis gravidarum, signs of hyperthyroidism, or uterine enlargement greater than expected for gestational age.

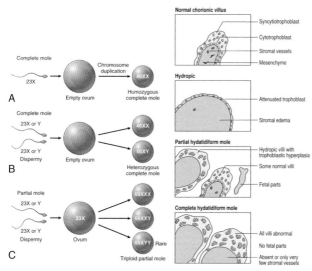

FIG. 5.28 Pathogenesis of molar pregnancies. (Modified [by Esther Baranov] from 2 images Elsevier Clinical Key: Figure 22.52. The female genital tract. Ellenson LH, Pirog EC: *Robbins and Cotran pathologic basis of disease*, Chapter 22, pp 991–1042. Figure 19.25. Female genital tract. Wells M: *Underwood's pathology: a clinical approach*, 19, pp 442–469.)

- Partial moles often present as missed abortions.
- Risk factors:
  - Prior molar pregnancy
  - Asian ethnicity
  - Multiparity
  - Prior spontaneous abortions

PPx: N/A

MoD: See Table 5.3

- **Complete moles** (diploid) are formed when two sperm fertilize an empty ovum (egg with no genetic material) or one sperm fertilizes an empty ovum and undergoes chromosomal duplication. This aberrant fertilization produces an unviable pregnancy and a neoplasm capable of malignant transformation and local invasion.
- **Partial moles** (triploid) are formed when two sperm fertilize an ovum (with retained genetic material), also producing an unviable pregnancy and a neoplasm capable of malignant transformation and local invasion.

Dx:

1. Complete mole: Fig. 5.29
   - Serum β-hCG markedly elevated (often >100,000 mIU/mL).
   - TVUS → heterogeneous mass of multiple small hypoechoic areas resembling a "bunch of grapes" or a "snowstorm," absent fetal parts, absent

TABLE 5.3 Distinctions Between Complete and Partial Molar Pregnancies

Complete Hydatidiform Mole	Partial Hydatidiform Mole
46 XX, 46 XY **(diploid)**	69XXX, 69XXY, 69XYY **(triploid)**
1 sperm (with chromosomal duplication) or 2 sperm fertilize an *empty* ovum	2 sperm fertilize an ovum *with genetic material*
Absent fetus (absent fetal heart sounds)	Fetus or fetal parts often present
Absent amnion	Amnion/fetal red blood cells usually present
Diffuse villous edema and trophoblastic proliferation	Focal and variable villous edema, focal trophoblastic proliferation
Usually diagnosed as a molar pregnancy on routine ultrasound, may present with spontaneous abortion (vaginal bleeding and passage of hydropic vesicles)	Usually initially diagnosed as a missed abortion
Classic "snowstorm" appearance on TVUS	Focal abnormalities may be seen on TVUS but generally difficult to dx via ultrasound
Associated with hyperemesis gravidarum, early preeclampsia, hyperthyroidism, and multiple theca lutein cysts due to excess β-hCG	Not typically associated with as many systemic symptoms as β-hCG levels are often normal or only slightly elevated
Uterine size often large for gestational age	Uterine size often small for gestational age
Up to a third develop malignant sequelae	Rarely develop malignant sequelae (5%)

hCG, Human chorionic gonadotropin; *TVUS,* transvaginal ultrasound.

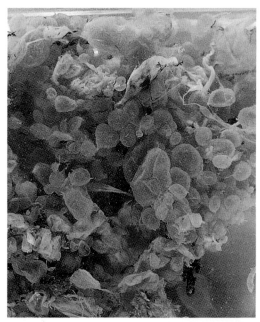

FIG. 5.29 Gross pathology image of a complete hydatidiform mole. (Modified [by Esther Baranov] from Elsevier Clinical Key: Figure 19.24. Female genital tract. Wells M: *Underwood's pathology: a clinical approach*, 19, pp 442–469.)

amniotic fluid, and absent vascularity on Doppler. Ovarian theca lutein cysts may also be visualized on TVUS.
- Final diagnosis is confirmed by histologic evaluation of the surgical specimen.

2. Partial mole:
   - Serum β-hCG normal or slightly elevated.
   - TVUS → focal placental abnormalities may be seen such as enlarged cystic anechoic areas, a growth-restricted fetus or fetal parts, and reduced amniotic fluid volume. However, partial moles are much harder to detect via ultrasound and are often misdiagnosed as missed abortions initially.
   - Final diagnosis is confirmed by histologic evaluation of the surgical specimen.

Tx/Mgmt:

1. **If a woman has not completed childbearing** → immediate evacuation with suction dilation and curettage (D&C).
2. **If a woman has completed childbearing** → hysterectomy recommended (decrease the risk of developing gestational trophoblastic neoplasia (GTN) following a molar pregnancy).
3. **If patient has dyspnea** → chest x-ray (CXR) for detection of early pulmonary metastases of GTN. More likely in complete moles.
4. **After D&E or hysterectomy** → follow-up with serial serum β-hCG monitoring and pelvic exams. ACOG (American College of Obstetricians and Gynecologists) recommends checking serum β-hCG within 48 hours after evacuation/hysterectomy, every week until they are not detectable for 3 weeks, followed by every month for an additional 6 months. If the serum β-hCG level remains undetectable throughout this time period, the patient may resume efforts to become pregnant. During the entire period of β-hCG surveillance, the patient must be counseled to use reliable methods of contraception.
5. **In high-risk patients or in patients unlikely to follow up with serial serum β-hCG monitoring** → chemoprophylaxis with methotrexate or dactinomycin to reduce the risk of developing GTN after a molar pregnancy.
6. Symptoms related to excessively high serum β-hCG, such as ovarian theca lutein cysts, hyperthyroidism, and preeclampsia, will all resolve with complete evacuation of the molar pregnancy and do not typically require additional treatment.

Gestational Trophoblastic Neoplasia

gg AR

Gestational trophoblastic neoplasia, APGO video

GTN is a diverse group of malignant neoplasms that arise from an abnormal proliferation of placental tropho-blasts. These neoplasms can occur following molar or nonmolar pregnancies (full term, preterm, spontaneous abortions, ectopic pregnancies), but molar pregnancies precede GTN approximately 50% of the time. These malignancies can arise months to years after a preg-nancy, sometimes making them quite difficult to recog-nize and diagnose.

Following evacuation of a hydatidiform mole, if serum β-hCG levels continue to rise or remain elevated over several weeks, the patient is classified as having GTN and requires treatment. AUB more than 6 weeks after a pregnancy of any kind should be evaluated with serum β-hCG and a pelvic ultrasound to exclude GTN. Likewise, metastases without a known primary in a woman of reproductive age should always be evaluated with a serum β-hCG level. In fact, a high serum hCG and exclusion of pregnancy are all that is required to diagnose metastatic GTN in these circumstances.

Definition: There are four distinct varieties of GTN as outlined below:

Buzz Words: Lung or vaginal metastases + lesions on CXR in a recently pregnant woman + rising serum β-hCG after pregnancy + AUB <6 months after pregnancy

Clinical Presentation:

- **Invasive mole** → present after evacuation of hydatidi-form mole with persistently elevated serum β-hCG, vaginal bleeding, enlarged uterus, pelvic pressure/pain, and theca lutein cysts.
- **Gestational choriocarcinoma** → present months to years after molar or nonmolar pregnancy with **extremely elevated serum β-hCG**, vaginal bleeding, pelvic pressure/pain, theca lutein cysts, hyperthyroid-ism, and symptoms related to metastases (*lung mets*—shortness of breath, chest pain, cough, hemoptysis; *brain mets*—headaches, dizziness, seizures; *liver or GI mets*—abdominal pain, melena) (Fig. 5.30)
- Risk factors include: advanced maternal age, prior molar pregnancy, Asian ethnicity

PPx: N/A

MoD: Due to dysfunctional imprinting because paternal genes are known to control placental growth, whereas maternal genes control fetal growth. Excess paternal genetic material, as in hydatidiform moles, leads to excessive placental trophoblastic proliferation.

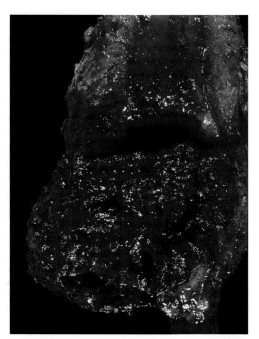

FIG. 5.30 Gross pathology image of choriocarcinoma, seen here as a hemorrhagic mass filling the uterine cavity. (Modified [by Esther Baranov] from Elsevier Clinical Key: Figure 13C.16. Tumors of the female genital tract. Fletcher CDM: *Diagnostic histopathology of tumors*, Chapter 13, pp 658–871.)

Dx:

1. GTN is ultimately a clinical diagnosis, based on history, physical exam, imaging, and serum ß-hCG. Below are the appropriate diagnostic steps when GTN is suspected:
   - **Serum β-hCG determination** → an elevated serum β-hCG is required for the diagnosis for GTN, and an extremely elevated β-hCG (>100,000 mIU/mL) is virtually diagnostic:
     - Dx after evacuation of a molar pregnancy (serial β-hCG monitoring): if weekly serum β-hCG levels plateau over 3 weeks, if β-hCG levels increase more than 10% over a 2-week duration (3 values), or if serum β-hCG levels are detectable for greater than 6 months, a diagnosis of GTN is made and treatment is initiated.
   - **Pelvic speculum exam** → to look for vaginal metastases, however, these highly vascular lesions should not be biopsied and uterine curettage should not be attempted, as there is a risk for severe hemorrhage.
   - **Pelvic ultrasound** → to evaluate for viable pregnancy or evidence of GTN, which can be seen on TVUS as a heterogeneous, hyperechoic, cystic mass within

the myometrium with prominent hypervascularity on Doppler and no evidence of a fetus. Enlarged ovaries can also be seen with GTN, due to bilateral theca lutein cysts from β-hCG hyperstimulation (more common with invasive mole and choriocarcinoma).

- **CXR (or CT Chest)** → to determine if lung metastases are present.
- **CT head, CT A/P** → if CXR/CT is positive for lung lesions, then imaging (either CT/MRI) of brain and abdomen/pelvis is warranted to look for brain or liver metastases.
- Final definitive diagnosis is confirmed by histologic evaluation of the surgical specimen if hysterectomy is performed.

Tx/Mgmt:

1. GTN has an almost 100% survival with appropriate treatment and early detection.
   - **Invasive mole** → initiate single-agent chemotherapy (methotrexate or dactinomycin) and continue β-hCG monitoring. Avoid D&C so as not to cause uterine perforation.
   - **Gestational choriocarcinoma without metastases** → initiate single-agent chemotherapy (methotrexate or dactinomycin) and continue β-hCG monitoring.
   - **Gestational choriocarcinoma with metastases** → initiate chemotherapy as soon as possible because bleeding complications from metastases (especially in the brain) can be fatal:
     - If patient is low-risk → single-agent chemotherapy can be used; typically methotrexate or dactinomycin.
     - If patient is high-risk → multiagent chemotherapy required; typically triple therapy with methotrexate, dactinomycin, and either cyclophosphamide or chlorambucil.
     - Patients with metastatic gestational choriocarcinoma are considered high-risk if they have any one of the following features:
       - Preceding molar pregnancy with extremely high serum β-hCG (>100,000 mIU/mL)
       - Advanced maternal age (>39)
       - Liver or brain metastases
       - >4 months since prior pregnancy
       - Pregnancy preceding GTN was a term pregnancy
       - Failure of a single chemotherapy agent
   - Hysterectomy is appropriate treatment for patients with GTN who are older and do not desire future

TABLE 5.4 Distinctions Between Invasive Mole, Gestational Choriocarcinoma, Placental Site Trophoblastic Tumor, and Epithelioid Trophoblastic Tumor

	Definition	Characteristics	Behavior
Invasive mole	Abnormal trophoblastic proliferation characterized by edematous chorionic villi invading directly into the uterine myometrium	Occur exclusively after a molar pregnancy (complete or partial); elevated serum β-hCG	Can be confined to uterus or locally invasive, invading into peritoneum or vaginal vault. Vascular invasion and metastases occur very rarely. Usually present <6 months after molar pregnancy.
Gestational choriocarcinoma (GC)	Abnormal proliferation of anaplastic mononucleated cytotrophoblasts and multinucleated syncytiotrophoblasts (no chorionic villi)	Most prevalent GTN overall; often occur after a molar pregnancy, particularly a complete mole; extremely elevated serum β-hCG	Early vascular invasion, with metastases to lungs, vagina, liver, and brain due to hematogenous spread. Typically diagnosed when already metastatic.
Placental site trophoblastic tumor (PSTT)[a]	Abnormal proliferation of placental intermediate trophoblasts (no chorionic villi)	Rare; more commonly occur after non-molar pregnancy or abortion; relatively low levels of serum β-hCG compared to GC	Can present several years after gestational event. Disease confined to uterus for many years. Patients often present late due to lack of obvious symptoms.
Epithelioid trophoblastic tumor[a]	Abnormal proliferation of placental intermediate trophoblasts (no chorionic villi)	Extremely rare variant of PSTT; relatively low levels of serum β-hCG compared to GC	Disease confined to the uterus for many years. Patients often present late due to lack of obvious symptoms.

[a]**Note**: PSTT and ETT are very rare entities and are unlikely to be on your shelf exam or even come up on your clinical rotations. They are added here for sake of completion, but you should focus most your attention on invasive moles and gestational choriocarcinoma as these are far more common and are important to recognize.
GTN, Gestational trophoblastic neoplasia; *hCG*, Human chorionic gonadotropin.

childbirth, who are resistant to chemotherapy, or who are poorly compliant.

- Weekly serial β-hCG monitoring is required for all GTN while levels remain elevated, followed by monthly β-hCG monitoring for 12 months once complete resolution of serum β-hCG levels is achieved (Table 5.4).

Uterine Leiomyosarcoma

Definition: Rare, aggressive, malignant smooth muscle tumor that arises in the uterine myometrium and carries a poor prognosis with an extremely high recurrence rate even for early-stage disease (70% recurrence in stage I and II).

Buzz Words: Rapidly enlarging pelvic mass + postmenopausal woman + AUB + pelvic pain

Clinical Presentation: Leiomyosarcomas present similarly to uterine leiomyomas, with AUB, pelvic pain/pressure, urinary symptoms, constipation. However, a rapidly enlarging pelvic mass should be suspicious for a sarcoma. Risk factors include African American ethnicity, prior tamoxifen therapy, or pelvic radiation.

PPx: N/A

MoD: Leiomyosarcomas are NOT believed to arise from leiomyomas. Leiomyosarcomas are often quite large (>10 cm) and poorly circumscribed, classically displaying areas of hemorrhage and necrosis. They spread hematogenously, most commonly metastasizing to the lungs and liver. Histology of these neoplasms reveals prominent cellular and nuclear atypia and numerous mitoses per high power field (HPF) (high mitotic index). Cytogenetics reveal frequent aneuploidy and complex karyotypes with multiple chromosomal abnormalities.

Dx:

1. Diagnosis of uterine leiomyosarcoma is often made after surgery for a preoperative diagnosis of uterine leiomyomas (fibroids).
2. The final diagnosis is confirmed by histologic evaluation of the surgical specimen:
   - Histologically, a smooth muscle tumor is classified as a leiomyosarcoma if the following criteria are present:
     - Moderate-to-severe cytologic atypia
     - Greater than 5 mitoses per 10 HPFs
     - Tumor cell necrosis

Tx/Mgmt:

1. Imaging (CXR, CT, and/or MRI) to determine the presence of metastases at the time of diagnosis.
2. Benefit of adjuvant chemotherapy or radiotherapy on overall survival in patients with leiomyosarcoma remains controversial.
3. Palliative surgery may be performed for patients experiencing significant pain or vaginal bleeding secondary to the uterine mass.
4. FIGO staging for leiomyosarcomas differs from staging for EC, and importantly, staging does not predict prognosis for overall survival as well as it does for many other cancers.

Benign Neoplasms and Cysts of the Cervix

Nabothian Cyst

Buzz Words: "Epithelial inclusion cyst" + "mucinous retention cyst" + cervical cyst + asymptomatic

Clinical Presentation: Found in reproductive-aged women who are mostly asymptomatic. Can present with pain,

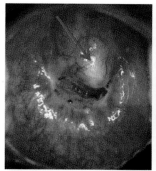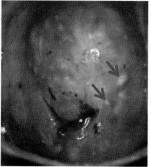

FIG. 5.31 Nabothian cysts *(yellow arrows)*, as seen at colposcopy. Note that one cervix has a single large nabothian cyst, whereas the other has numerous small nabothian cysts (only some of which are highlighted with *arrows*). (Modified by Esther Baranov from [2 images] Elsevier Clinical Key: Plate 7.1. Normal transformation zone. O'Connor DM. *Colposcopy*, Chapter 7, pp 125–142; and Figure 9.1. Abnormal transformation zone. Brotzman GL, Apgar BS. *Colposcopy*, Chapter 9, pp 149–163.)

irritation, dyspareunia (pain during sexual intercourse), or a sensation of pressure (Fig. 5.31).

PPx: N/A

MoD: Squamous epithelium grows over a small crevice of secretory columnar epithelium (gland crypt) that continues to secrete mucinous material, forming a simple cyst.

Dx:
1. Clinical diagnosis made by visualization through a speculum.

Tx/Mgmt:
1. Treat only if symptomatic, with either electrocautery ablation or surgical excision (if concerning for malignancy).

Endocervical Polyp

Definition: Beefy-red, glistening, vascular masses that arise from the endocervical canal and protrude through the external cervical os.

Buzz Words: Postcoital spotting + vaginal bleeding

Clinical Presentation: A reproductive-aged women, especially >40 years, reports postcoital spotting and vaginal bleeding/discharge between menses (Fig. 5.32).

PPx: N/A

MoD: Unknown

Dx:
1. Visualized as a beefy-red polyp protruding through cervical os on speculum exam.

Tx/Mgmt:
1. Polypectomy is performed if polyp is symptomatic, larger than 3 cm, or appears atypical.
2. Malignancy is exceedingly rare in cervical polyps.

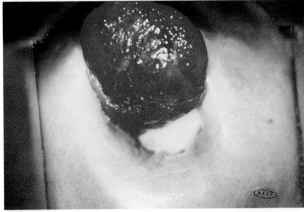

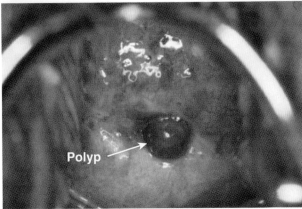

FIG. 5.32 Two endocervical polyps of different sizes seen as beefy-red masses protruding through the cervical os on speculum exam. (Modified [by Esther Baranov] from 2 images Elsevier Clinical Key: Figure 18.22. Benign gynecologic lesions. Dolan MS, Hill C, Valea FA: *Comprehensive gynecology*, 18, pp 370–422.e5; and Figure 137.4. Colposcopic examination. Newkirk GR: *Pfenninger and Fowler's procedures for primary care*, Chapter 137, pp 919–935.)

Malignant and Premalignant Neoplasms of the Cervix

Cervical Dysplasia and Management of Abnormal Pap Smears

Definitions:

- **Cervical dysplasia** = atypical cellular change within the cervical squamous epithelium due to persistent HPV infection and active replication of the virus.
- **Human papillomavirus** = a DNA virus with numerous distinct genotypes of differing oncogenic potential and tropism for epithelium of the cervix, vagina, vulva, anus, and oropharynx.

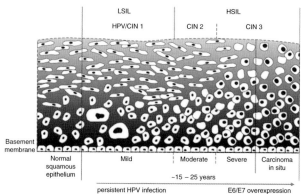

FIG. 5.33 Diagram showing progressive stages of cervical dysplasia over time, eventually involving the full thickness of the cervical epithelium as nuclei become larger and more irregularly shaped. *CIN*, Cervical intraepithelial neoplasia; *HSIL*, high-grade squamous intraepithelial lesion; *HPV*, human papillomavirus; *LSIL*, low-grade squamous intraepithelial lesion. (Modified by Esther Baranov from Figure 28.4. Intraepithelial neoplasia of the lower genital tract [cervix, vagina, vulva]. Salcedo MP, Baker ES, Schmeler KM: *Comprehensive gynecology*, 28, pp 655–665.)

- **Cervical intraepithelial neoplasia (CIN)** = premalignant dysplasia of cervical squamous epithelium, which encompasses the lower third (CIN 1), lower two-thirds (CIN 2), or greater than two-thirds (CIN 3) of the epithelial thickness. This terminology was used to classify premalignant cervical dysplasia prior to 2012, with the degree of dysplasia (mild, moderate, or severe) increasing from CIN 1 to CIN 3 (Fig. 5.33).
- **Atypical squamous cells of undetermined significance (ASC-US)** = squamous cells seen on cervical cytology specimens (Pap smears) that differ from normal epithelial cells but do not meet criteria for a squamous intraepithelial lesion.
- **Low-grade squamous intraepithelial lesion (LSIL)** = on cervical cytology, squamous cells with mild dysplastic changes such as koilocytosis, nuclear enlargement, and hyperchromasia. On histology (biopsy), a low-grade lesion with mild dysplasia of the lower third of the cervical epithelium (CIN 1) or dysplasia of the lower two-thirds of the epithelium (CIN 2) that is negative for p16 by immunohistochemistry.
- **High-grade squamous intraepithelial lesion (HSIL)** = on cervical cytology, squamous cells with moderate-to-severe dysplasia. On histology, a high-grade lesion (CIN 3) with dysplasia of two-thirds to full thickness of the cervical epithelium, often with markedly dysplastic cells. HSIL also refers to lesions with dysplasia encompassing

AR

Cervical Screening Guidlines, USPSTF

QUICK TIP

Immunohistochemical (IHC) staining for p16 overexpression is used as a surrogate marker for HPV viral protein E6/E7 activity, which is suggestive of a higher-grade lesion that will more likely progress to cervical carcinoma.

two-thirds of the epithelium (previously CIN 2) that are positive for p16 by immunohistochemistry.

- **Atypical squamous cells, cannot exclude high-grade squamous intraepithelial lesion (ASC-H)** = squamous cells seen on cervical cytology that display abnormalities suspicious for HSIL and likely are a mixture of true HSIL and other findings that could mimic HSIL. This cytology finding is associated with a much higher risk of cervical neoplasia than ASC-US.
- **Atypical glandular cells (AGC)** = require further investigation.
- **"Co-testing"** = simultaneous cervical cytology (Pap smear) examination and high-risk HPV DNA testing performed on the same cervical sample to improve detection of cervical neoplasia. Co-testing is recommended for women after the age of 29.
- **Reflex HPV testing** = testing for high-risk HPV DNA performed on the same cervical sample used for cytology *only* if results reveal ASC-US. Reflex HPV testing is recommended for women ages 25–29.

Buzz Words: Abnormal Pap smears + history of STIs + sexually active, acetowhite changes on colposcopy + post-coital spotting

Clinical Presentation:
- Age: 21–65, no testing for HPV or cervical dysplasia recommended prior to 21 or after 65 (if patient has no history of positive Pap smears and is up to date with screening).
- Risk factors: Most are related to an increased risk of infection with HPV, namely increased or early onset of sexual intercourse:
  - Young age at first sexual intercourse
  - Multiple sexual partners
  - Sexual intercourse with high-risk partners (partners who have had multiple sexual partners)
  - History of STIs
  - History of vulvar or vaginal squamous dysplasia or cancer (also caused by HPV infection)
  - Early age at first childbirth
  - Multiparity
  - Low socioeconomic status
  - Cigarette smoking (associated with cervical SCC but not adenocarcinoma)

PPx: HPV vaccination prior to initiation of sexual activity can prevent infection with HPV 6, 11, 16, 18. The recommendations for cervical cancer screening in vaccinated women are the *same* as unvaccinated women.

MoD: Infection of cervical squamous epithelium with HPV → persistence of HPV infection (likelihood of persistence higher in older women, immunosuppressed women, or those infected with high-risk HPV genotypes) → active viral replication causes dysplasia seen on cervical cytology → HPV is eventually cleared or HPV integrates its genome with host DNA causing overexpression of E6/E7 viral oncogenes in cervical epithelium → HSIL → invasive cervical carcinoma.

Dx:

1. **Cervical cytology (Pap smear)** = a screening tool used to assess for premalignant cervical dysplasia or cancer by microscopic evaluation of cytologic features in cells that are scraped off the cervix and endocervical canal during a speculum examination.
2. **Colposcopy** = a procedure involving a microscope (colposcope) to directly visualize the cervix with higher magnification and take biopsies of any suspicious areas, usually performed when a Pap smear reveals abnormal or undetermined cytology. During colposcopy, the physician will apply acetic acid to the cervix, which dries out the dysplastic cells more than the normal cells and highlights dysplasia as acetowhite changes (Figs. 5.34 and 5.35).

Tx/Mgmt:

1. **Normal cytology:**
   * **Women ages 21–24:** Cytology (Pap smear) every 3 years
   * **Women ages 25–29:** Cytology every 3 years with reflex testing for HPV

> **QUICK TIP**
>
> HPV genotypes 16 and 18 are most commonly isolated from HSIL and cervical cancer specimens and are thus designated high-risk (oncogenic) HPV genotypes, in contrast to genotypes 6 and 11, which are most often isolated from anogenital warts or LSIL and are designated low-risk (low oncogenic potential).

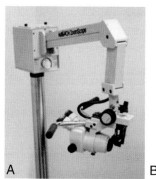
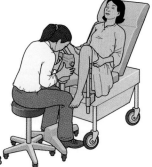

FIG. 5.34 Image of a colposcope (A) and illustration of a gynecologist visualizing the cervix through a colposcope. (From Elsevier Clinical Key: Figure 58.8. Examination of the sexual assault victim. Sachs CJ, Wheeler M: *Roberts and Hedges' clinical procedures in emergency medicine*, Chapter 58, pp 1188–1203.e1.)

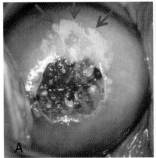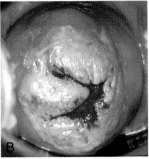

FIG. 5.35 Colposcopy images revealing a lesion of acetowhite epithelium with geographic borders between 11 and 2 o'clock suggestive of a high-grade squamous intraepithelial lesion (A, *yellow arrows*) and a circumferential lesion of thick acetowhite epithelium with a coarse mosaic pattern suggestive of a low-grade squamous intraepithelial lesion (B). (Modified by Esther Baranov from [2 images] Elsevier Clinical Key: Figure 12.8. Low-grade squamous intraepithelial lesions. Waxman AG: *Colposcopy*, Chapter 12, pp 201–230; and Figure 13.10. High-grade squamous intraepithelial lesions. Massad LS: *Colposcopy*, Chapter 13, pp 231–260.)

- **Women ages 30 and above:** Co-testing with HPV is preferred, but cytology every 3 years with reflex testing for HPV is an acceptable alternative.
2. ASC-US cytology:
   - **Women ages 21–24 with ASC-US cytology:** Repeat cytology in 12 months. HPV reflex testing is not advised in this age group because risk of cervical cancer is low, risk of HPV infection is high, and the majority of cervical dysplasia in this age group regresses spontaneously.
   - **Women ages 25–29 with ASC-US cytology:** HPV reflex testing is recommended in this age group, but repeat cytology in 12 months is also acceptable:
     - If HPV reflex testing is negative → co-testing in 3 years
     - If HPV reflex testing positive → colposcopy
   - **Women age 30 and above:** HPV co-testing every 5 years is recommended for cervical cancer screening in this group. Cytology every 3 years with HPV reflex testing for ASC-US results is also acceptable.
   - If negative for HPV with ASC-US cytology → co-testing in 3 years (vs. co-testing in 5 years if cytology normal and HPV negative).
   - If positive for HPV with ASC-US cytology → colposcopy.
3. ASC-H cytology: All women with ASC-H should be evaluated with colposcopy. Note that immediate

loop electrosurgical excision procedure (LEEP) is not appropriate.
4. LSIL:
   - If high-risk strain HPV positive → colposcopy
   - If HPV negative → Pap test and HPV testing in 1 year
5. HSIL:
   - Age 21–24 or pregnant → colposcopy
   - All others → proceed to LEEP

Cervical Cancer

In the United States and other developed countries of the world, cervical cancer has the third highest incidence and mortality rate among gynecologic malignancies, after endometrial and ovarian cancers. However, in developing and underdeveloped nations, cervical cancer has the second highest incidence and mortality rate among *all* malignancies in women, largely due to inadequate vaccination against HPV and insufficient screening. In Africa and Central America, cervical cancer is the number one cause of death by cancer among women.

Importantly, HPV can be detected in 99.7% of all cervical cancers, suggesting an inextricable link between infection with HPV and development of cervical cancer. In fact, recent studies have shown significant drops in rates of high-grade cervical dysplasia in areas where HPV vaccination rates have increased, suggesting cervical cancer incidence in these areas will likely decrease as well. This underscores the importance of HPV vaccination in preventing the development of cervical dysplasia and cancer.

Cervical cancer can be broken down into two main histological subtypes, SCC (70%) and adenocarcinoma (25%), with the remainder comprised of less common cervical cancer variants (e.g., adenosquamous, adenoid cystic, undifferentiated). Unlike ovarian and ECs, which are staged surgically, cervical cancer is staged *clinically* (Table 5.5) by information obtained from a bimanual pelvic examination and rectal-vaginal examination as well as colposcopy, cystoscopy, proctosigmoidoscopy, x-ray, barium enema, or intravenous pyelogram depending on the patient's clinical presentation. Radioimaging modalities such as CT, TVUS, and MRI are not used to stage cervical cancer but can be clinically useful for surgical planning.

Buzz Words: Malodorous vaginal discharge + abnormal vaginal bleeding + exophytic cervical lesion + history of abnormal Pap smears + lost to follow-up + nonadherence to cervical cancer screening guidelines

TABLE 5.5 International Federation of Gynecology and Obstetrics 2009 Staging for Cervical Cancer[a]

Stage	Extent of Disease	5-Year Survival
I	Tumor limited to uterus	~75%–98%
IA	Microscopic stromal invasion of ≤3 mm depth, ≤7 mm width (IA1) or >3 mm but ≤5 mm depth, ≤7 mm width (IA2)	
IB	Clinically visible invasive tumor ≤4 cm (IB1) or >4 cm (IB2) in greatest dimension or microscopic stromal invasion >stage IA	
II	Tumor limited to upper two-thirds of vagina and/or parametria	~65%–75%
IIA	Extension to upper two-thirds of vagina with tumor ≤4 cm (IIA1) or >4 cm (IIA2) in greatest dimension	
IIB	Parametrial invasion of tumor	
III	Tumor limited to vagina and pelvic wall ± hydronephrosis	~40%–45%
IIIA	Extension to lower third of vagina	
IIIB	Extension to pelvic sidewall and/or hydronephrosis or nonfunctioning kidney with no other explanation	
IV	Tumor invasion of bladder/bowel or distant metastases	~10%–20%
IVA	Invasion of bladder/bowel mucosa or adjacent pelvic organs	
IVB	Distant metastases to intra- or extra-abdominal organs (including peritoneal spread and/or para-aortic lymph nodes)	

[a]Details such as subdivisions of stage IA and IB are stated here for completion, but are ultimately low-yield in terms of examinations.

Clinical Presentation:

- Age: 30–85, mean age 48
- Chief Complaint: Postcoital spotting, abnormal vaginal bleeding, malodorous vaginal discharge (due to necrotic tumor), flank tenderness (hydronephrosis caused by tumor invasion into a ureter), constipation (tumor invasion into large bowel).
- Factors associated with progression to cervical cancer:
  - Oral contraceptive use (risk of invasive cervical cancer increases with duration of use, cause unknown)
  - Immunosuppressive therapy (less likely to clear HPV infections)
  - HIV (higher likelihood of infection with oncogenic HPV genotype and less likely to clear infection due to immunosuppression)
- Risk factors are equivalent to those for cervical dysplasia and are associated with an increased risk of exposure to HPV (see above).

PPx: HPV vaccination is primary prevention against cervical cancer, while screening for cervical dysplasia (Pap smears) is secondary prevention. Often, women who present with cervical cancer in the United States, especially later stages, have been lost to follow-up or noncompliant with regular cervical cancer screening, and therefore were not treated at earlier stages of cervical dysplasia (LSIL or HSIL).

MoD: ~15–25 years from initial infection with HPV to invasive carcinoma (Fig. 5.36).

- **HPV infection of cervical epithelium by oncogenic subtype** (e.g., genotypes 16, 18, 31, 33, 45, 58)— cervical cancer pathogenesis requires infection of the cervical epithelium by an oncogenic strain of HPV. HPV infects the basal epithelial cells through an abrasion in the cervical mucosa.
- **HPV persistence and replication in the cervical epithelium**—viral persistence and replication cause the infected epithelial cells to accumulate genetic mutations, leading to chromosomal instability, cell immortality, dysplasia, and eventually invasion through the basement membrane to form carcinoma.
- **HPV viral genome integration into the host genome and overexpression of oncogenes E6 and E7**—two of the six early (E) proteins encoded by the HPV viral genome (Fig. 5.37), viral oncogenes E6 and E7 are known to be central to cervical cancer pathogenesis (Fig. 5.38). E6 binds the cell cycle regulatory protein p53, which normally controls cell progression through the G1 checkpoint and triggers apoptosis if DNA damage is severe. Binding of E6 to p53 leads to its degradation, allowing for uninhibited cell replication and accumulation of unchecked DNA mutations. E7 binds and inhibits Rb, a protein that prevents cells from entering S phase with damaged DNA.
- **Overexpression of p16 as a marker of E6 and E7 integration into the host genome**—p16 is a tumor suppressor, which normally inhibits Rb and is kept at a basal level of expression by negative feedback from Rb. Once the HPV viral genome has been integrated into the host genome and the oncoproteins E6 and E7 are overexpressed, E7 readily binds to Rb. With Rb no longer providing negative feedback, p16 overexpression can be seen in the malignant lesion.

Dx:

1. Cervical biopsy if a suspicious cervical lesion is visualized on speculum exam or colposcopy (Fig. 5.39)
2. Cervical cytology (Pap smear) is not appropriate for *diagnosing* cervical cancer and can be used only for screening purposes.
3. Radioimaging modalities such as CT, TVUS, and MRI are not used to stage cervical cancer but can be clinically useful for surgical planning.

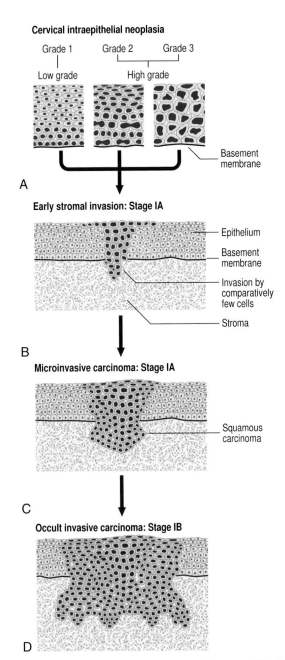

FIG. 5.36 Schematic image of early-stage cervical cancer. (Modified by Esther Baranov from Elsevier Clinical Key: Figure 19.7. Female genital tract. Wells M: *Underwood's pathology: a clinical approach*, 19, pp 442–469.)

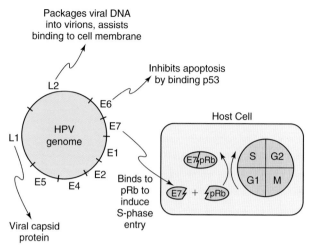

FIG. 5.37 Human papillomavirus (HPV) viral genome containing oncogenes E6 and E7, important in cervical cancer pathogenesis. (Modified by Esther Baranov from Elsevier Clinical Key: Figure 1.34. Cervical and vaginal cytology. Cibas ES. *Cytology*, Chapter 1, pp 1–57.)

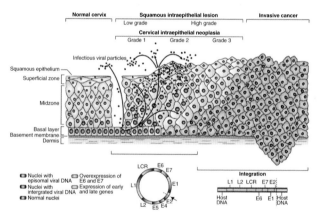

FIG. 5.38 Viral pathogenesis of cervical cancer. Note that initial human papillomavirus infection occurs through an abrasion in the epithelium to infect basal cells. Also note that low-grade dysplasia involves replication of viral episomal DNA with shedding of infectious particles, whereas high-grade dysplasia and invasive carcinoma require integration of the viral genome into the host DNA, causing overexpression of oncoproteins E6 and E7. (From Elsevier Clinical Key: Figure 2. Crosbie EJ, Einstein MH, Franceschi S, Kitchener HC: Human papillomavirus and cervical cancer. *Lancet* 382[9895]:889–899, 2013.)

Tx/Mgmt:

1. **Early-stage cervical cancer (stage I)** → modified radical hysterectomy (upper third of vagina is resected with uterus and cervix) with pelvic lymphadenectomy for definitive treatment. Patients with intermediate-risk or high-risk factors require adjuvant radiation therapy

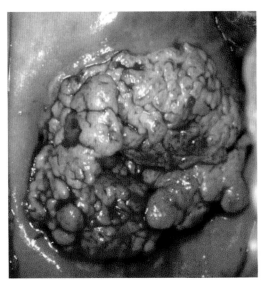

FIG. 5.39 Colposcopy image of cervical squamous cell carcinoma, revealing a friable, necrotic mass with atypical surface vasculature. (From Elsevier Clinical Key: Plates 14.11 and 14.14. Squamous cervical cancer. Reynolds RK. *Colposcopy*, Chapter 14, pp 261–282.)

or chemoradiation, respectively. Primary radiotherapy (RT) is acceptable if the patient is not a good surgical candidate.

2. **Early-stage cervical cancer and wish to pursue future childbearing** → fertility-sparing surgery if appropriate candidates with early-stage disease.
3. **Stage IA1 with no high-risk factors** → can undergo cone biopsy or extrafascial hysterectomy instead of modified radical hysterectomy if no high-risk factors.
4. **Locally advanced cervical cancer (stage IB2 to IVA)** → primary chemoradiation (with cisplatin) during radiation therapy. Surgery is not likely to be curative in these patients and is not offered.

Benign Neoplasms and Cysts of the Vagina and Vulva

Gartner Duct Cyst

Definition: Common vaginal mass found along the anterior and lateral vaginal walls that forms due to cystic dilation of an obstructed Gartner duct.

Buzz Words: Asymptomatic vaginal mass, anterolateral wall

Clinical Presentation: A painless vaginal mass, it is often asymptomatic but can occasionally cause discomfort if large (Fig. 5.40).

PPx: N/A

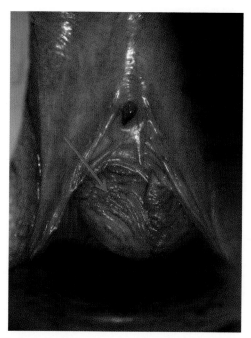

FIG. 5.40 Gartner duct cyst *(yellow arrow)* seen as an anterior vaginal wall mass just below the urethra. (Modified by Esther Baranov from Elsevier Clinical Key: Figure 11.3. Benign vaginal wall masses and paraurethral lesions. Shah SR, Nitti VW: *Vaginal surgery for the urologist*, 11, pp 127–135.)

MoD: Gartner ducts are remnants of the embryonic mesonephric (Wolffian) ducts that course over the anterolateral aspect of the vaginal canal. Cysts can arise in these ducts if they become obstructed, though they are typically small, asymptomatic, and incidentally found.

Dx:
1. Often an incidental finding on pelvic examination
2. Clinical diagnosis of finding a soft, painless vaginal mass along the anterior or lateral vaginal walls

Tx/Mgmt:
1. Surgical excision only if the cyst becomes symptomatic.

Vulvar Lichen Sclerosus

Definition: A chronic progressive inflammatory cutaneous condition of the vulva and anus characterized by thin, fragile, atrophic skin, architectural distortion of the vulva, pruritus, and often pain.

Buzz Words: "Porcelain-white" plaques + vulvar itching + dyspareunia + loss/fusion of labia minora + "cigarette paper" skin (fragile, thinned, atrophic wrinkled skin) + "figure-eight" pattern of affected skin around the anus and vulva (Fig. 5.41)

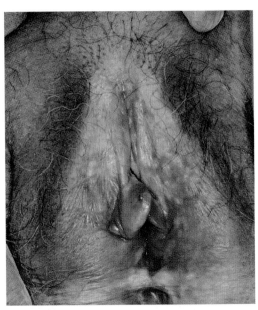

FIG. 5.41 Image of vulvar lichen sclerosus displaying the classic porcelain-white figure-eight pattern of affected skin around the anus and vulva with loss of the labia minora and evidence of inflammation. (Modified by Esther Baranov from Elsevier Clinical Key: eFigure 12.19. Lichen planus and related conditions. James WD, Berger TG, Elston DM: *Andrews' diseases of the skin*, 12, 209–224.e4.)

Clinical Presentation:
- Age: Prepubertal or postmenopausal women (bimodal age distribution)
- Chief Complaint: Vulvar pruritus, vulvar pain, dyspareunia, dysuria (especially with fusion of labia minora obstructing urethra), loss/fusion of labia minora (burying of clitoris behind clitoral hood), white atrophic papules and plaques, narrowing of vaginal introitus due to scarring
- PMH: More common in patients with autoimmune disease (thyroid disease, pernicious anemia, systemic lupus erythematosus)

PPx: N/A

MoD: Unknown

Dx:
1. Clinical diagnosis made by visualization of white plaques on a background of thin, wrinkled skin surrounding the vulva and/or anus, often with loss or fusion of the labia minora and marked architectural distortion in long-standing lesions.
2. Final diagnosis is confirmed by histologic evaluation of a vulvar punch biopsy specimen.

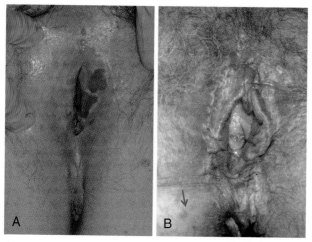

FIG. 5.42 Image of erosive vulvar lichen planus (A) with significant architectural distortion due to scarring, and papulosquamous vulvar lichen planus (B) with classic purple papules *(yellow arrow)* and lacy reticulate Wickham striae. (Modified by Esther Baranov from Elsevier Clinical Key: Figure 1. Lewis FM, Bogliatto F: Erosive vulval lichen planus—a diagnosis not to be missed: a clinical review. *Eur J Obstet Gynecol Reprod Biol* 171[2]:214–219, 2013, Copyright © 2013 Elsevier Ireland Ltd; and Figure 8.68. Psoriasis and other papulosquamous diseases. Habif TP: *Clinical dermatology*, Chapter 8, pp 263–328.)

Tx/Mgmt:
1. Topical corticosteroids (e.g., clobetasol propionate or halobetasol propionate)
2. Topical calcineurin inhibitors (e.g., tacrolimus) are second-line treatments, but can be used as steroid-sparing agents if significant cutaneous atrophy occurs.
3. Surveillance—5% risk of progression to vulvar SCC and patients should be examined yearly for suspicious lesions with biopsies performed on any hyperpigmented, indurated, fixed, or ulcerative lesions, or those that do not respond to treatment.

Vulvar Lichen Planus

Definition: Vulvar pain and pruritus with the presence of planar, purple, polygonal papules (papulosquamous variant) or erythematous mucosal erosions with white striae (erosive variant). Erosive vulvar lichen planus, which often involves the vagina as well, is the most severe form and can result in marked architectural destruction, including loss of the labia minora and narrowing of the vaginal introitus.

Buzz Words: Purple, polygonal, pruritic papules (papulosquamous variant) + erythematous mucosal lesions + Wickham striae (in erosive variant) (Fig. 5.42)

QUICK TIP

Remember the "5 Ps" of lichen planus—**p**ruritic, **p**lanar (flat), **p**urple, **p**olygonal, and **p**apular!

Clinical Presentation:
- Age: 50–60 years old
- Chief Complaint: Vulvar and vaginal pruritus, burning or pain, dyspareunia (vaginal stenosis), dysuria (urethral stenosis), vaginal discharge, severe vaginal synechiae (adhesions) leading to vaginal stenosis can occur with chronic lesions.
- PMH: More common in patients with autoimmune disease, often comorbid with cutaneous or oral lichen planus.

PPx: N/A

MoD: T-cell-mediated damage to basal keratinocytes in the epithelium.

Dx:
1. Clinical diagnosis made by visualization of purple polygonal papules or erythematous erosive mucosal lesions that classically contain reticular lacy white lines or borders called Wickham striae.
2. Final diagnosis is confirmed by histologic evaluation of a vulvar punch biopsy specimen.

QUICK TIP

Remember that lichen planus often involves the vagina, while lichen sclerosus rarely does, and that lichen sclerosus typically responds better to treatment.

Tx/Mgmt:
1. Topical corticosteroid ointments (e.g., clobetasol propionate)
2. Topical calcineurin inhibitors (e.g., tacrolimus)
3. Lesions are often resistant to therapy and systemic glucocorticoids or intralesional steroids may be required to get control over severe cases.
4. Maintenance—remission is possible, but there is no cure for lichen planus. Vaginal adhesions and scarring may require use of dilators or surgery for treatment.

Malignant and Premalignant Neoplasms of the Vagina and Vulva

Most primary neoplasms of the vagina and vulva are associated with infection by HPV (Table 5.6). Consequently, most of the risk factors for vulvar and vaginal SCC are related to an increased risk of infection with HPV and difficulty clearing the virus. Over 90% of vulvar carcinomas are vulvar SCC, which can be of two variants, classic type (associated with HPV) and differentiated type (associated with lichen sclerosus, not HPV). Primary vaginal cancer is quite rare and vaginal extension from other gynecological malignancies or metastases are far more common. As with vulvar carcinoma, most primary vaginal cancers are vaginal SCC (~85%). Although vaginal SCC is staged clinically, similar to cervical SCC, vulvar SCC is staged via a

TABLE 5.6 Clinical Lesions Associated With Human Papillomavirus Infection in Women

Benign Lesions
Condyloma acuminatum (anogenital wart)
Premalignant Lesions
Low-grade squamous intraepithelial lesion
High-grade squamous intraepithelial lesion
Vaginal intraepithelial neoplasia
Vulvar intraepithelial neoplasia
Anal intraepithelial neoplasia
Malignant Lesions
Invasive squamous cell carcinoma of the cervix
Invasive adenocarcinoma of the cervix
Invasive squamous cell carcinoma of the vagina
Invasive squamous cell carcinoma of the vulva
Invasive squamous cell carcinoma of the anus

combined clinical and surgical algorithm that considers inguinofemoral lymph node involvement and the extent of the vulvar lesion.

Condylomata Acuminata (Anogenital Warts)

Definition: Flesh-colored, cauliflower-like, papillary growths in the anogenital region with little to no malignant potential that develop because of infection by HPV, most frequently low-risk genotypes 6 and 11 (90% of anogenital warts) (Fig. 5.43).

Buzz Words: "Cauliflower-like" growth + anogenital + HPV genotypes 6 and 11

Clinical Presentation:
- Age: sexually active women
- Chief Complaint: Flesh-colored papillary growths on the vulva, vagina, cervix, or anus; most often asymptomatic, can present with pruritus, bleeding, burning, tenderness, or vaginal discharge
- Risk factors:
  - Immunosuppression
  - Increasing risk with number of sexual partners

PPx: HPV vaccination prior to initiation of sexual activity can prevent infection with a select number of HPV strains, including low-risk HPV genotypes 6 and 11, which cause most anogenital warts (90%).

MoD: Infection of the vulvar, vaginal, cervical, or anal squamous epithelium with low-risk HPV occurs via direct contact with infected individuals through vaginal intercourse or receptive anal intercourse. Persistence and replication

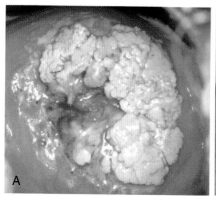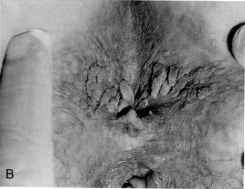

A   B

FIG. 5.43 Condylomata acuminata of the cervix (A) and vulva (B), displaying classic flesh-colored cauliflower-like growths. Note that the cervical condyloma could be mistaken for cervical carcinoma, however, there are no atypical surface vessels. (From Elsevier Clinical Key: Figure 12.7. Low-grade squamous intraepithelial lesions. Waxman AG: *Colposcopy*, Chapter 12, pp 201–230; and Figure 27.17. Viral infections. Ferri FF: *Ferri's color atlas and text of clinical medicine*, Chapter 27, pp 115–133.)

of the virus within the epithelium causes the cytologic changes that manifest as a papillary growth (Fig. 5.44).

Dx:
1. Clinical diagnosis by visual inspection.
2. Any suspicious, rapidly growing, or ulcerated lesions should be biopsied to determine if dysplasia or SCC is present.

Tx/Mgmt:
1. Asymptomatic anogenital warts require no intervention and may regress.
2. Topical agents typically used for larger areas (podophyllotoxin, podophyllin, trichloracetic acid, imiquimod).
3. Surgical excision/cryotherapy/laser ablation if symptomatic:
   - No therapy can eradicate every cell infected with HPV, leading to a relatively high rate of recurrence (20%–30%).
   - Although not believed to be premalignant lesions themselves, anogenital warts carry an increased risk of cervical and anogenital SCC because they mark exposure to HPV (exposure to one subtype of HPV indicates exposure to all subtypes of HPV, including high-risk genotypes).

Vulvar Intraepithelial Neoplasm and Vulvar Squamous Cell Carcinoma

Definition: Premalignant dysplasia (vulvar intraepithelial neoplasm [VIN]) or invasive carcinoma (SCC) of the vulvar

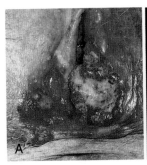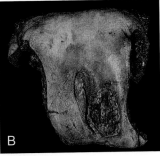

FIG. 5.44 Image of an ulcerated vulvar squamous cell carcinoma (A). Gross pathology image of a vulvectomy specimen for vulvar squamous cell carcinoma (B). (From Elsevier Clinical Key: Figure 20.2. Gynaecological oncology. Ngan HYS, Chan KKL: *Essential obstetrics and gynaecology*, Chapter 20, pp 317–339; and Figure 19.11. Female reproductive system. Rosai J: *Rosai & Ackerman's surgical pathology*, 19, pp 1399–1657.)

squamous epithelium that often occurs due to persistent infection with oncogenic subtypes of HPV, but can also occur as a result of chronic lichen sclerosus:

- **VIN/SCC, usual type**—associated with HPV infection (particularly genotypes 16, 18, 33); often presents in younger (premenopausal) women. The vast majority (90%) of VIN is related to HPV (usual type), but a lesser majority (60%) of vulvar SCC is related to HPV.
- **VIN/SCC, differentiated type**—associated with chronic inflammatory vulvar dystrophies (e.g., lichen sclerosus), not associated with HPV; often presents in older (postmenopausal) women as unifocal lesion. VIN, differentiated type, has a higher risk of progression to vulvar SCC and should always be excised.

Buzz Words: Chronic vulvar pruritus + vulvar lesion (nodule, plaque, or ulcer)

Clinical Presentation:

- Chief Complaint: Chronic vulvar pruritus, lesion(s) on labia majora, enlarged lymph node in groin, may also be asymptomatic.
- Risk factors for VIN and vulvar SCC are similar to those for cervical dysplasia and cancer (see above), and include cigarette smoking, vulvar dystrophy (e.g., lichen sclerosus), prior history of vulvar or cervical dysplasia, immunodeficiency (HIV), and northern European ancestry.

PPx:

- HPV vaccination prior to initiation of sexual activity
- Smoking cessation
- No routine screening for VIN or vulvar carcinoma

MoD: VIN/SCC, usual type carcinogenesis involves persistent infection with oncogenic HPV genotypes 16, 18, and 33, mechanism identical to cervical cancer; see above; differentiated type carcinogenesis is the result of chronic inflammation from long-standing lichen sclerosus (or other vulvar dystrophy).

Dx:

1. Histologic evaluation of a biopsy taken from the center of the suspicious vulvar lesion with final diagnosis confirmed on surgical excision specimen.

Tx/Mgmt:

1. VIN:
   - Wide local excision, partial vulvectomy, or laser ablation for smaller lesions
2. Vulvar SCC:
   - Surgical excision ± inguinofemoral lymphadenectomy, chemoradiation

Vaginal Intraepithelial Neoplasm and Vaginal Squamous Cell Carcinoma

Definition: Premalignant dysplasia (vaginal intraepithelial neoplasm [VAIN]) or invasive carcinoma (SCC) of the vaginal squamous epithelium that occurs as a result of persistent infection with oncogenic subtypes of HPV.

Buzz Words: Postcoital vaginal bleeding or PMB

Clinical Presentation:
- Age: postmenopausal women
- Chief Complaint: Vaginal bleeding, but may also present with malodorous vaginal discharge, vaginal mass, or be asymptomatic (malignancy detected via cervical cytology or on routine pelvic exam)
- Risk factors identical to those for cervical dysplasia, cervical cancer

PPx:
- HPV vaccination prior to initiation of sexual activity
- Smoking cessation
- No routine screening for VAIN or vaginal carcinoma

MoD: Persistent infection with oncogenic HPV genotypes, mechanism identical to cervical cancer; see above.

Dx:

1. Histologic evaluation of a biopsy from suspicious vaginal lesions with final diagnosis confirmed on surgical excision specimen.
2. The most common site for development of VAIN/vaginal SCC is the upper third of the posterior vaginal wall.

Tx/Mgmt:

1. VAIN is typically treated with local excision, partial or total vaginectomy.

2. May discover concomitant vulvar SCC undetected on biopsy (up to 25% of cases). Newer techniques involve CO_2 laser ablation as well as topical agents, but should only be used if there is no suspicion for invasive carcinoma. Recurrence rate is approximately 20%–30% with treatment.

3. Vaginal carcinoma, like cervical carcinoma, is staged clinically, requiring information obtained from a bimanual pelvic examination as well as colposcopy, cystoscopy, proctosigmoidoscopy, chest and skeletal x-ray:
   - Stage at time of diagnosis is the most important prognostic factor in vaginal cancer.

GUNNER PRACTICE

1. A 63-year-old woman presents to her primary care doctor with complaints of fatigue, loss of appetite, early satiety, some vague abdominal discomfort, and urinary urgency. She has not been feeling well lately, has been having some difficulty breathing, and thinks she may have even lost some weight. Her physician does a full physical exam as well as a pelvic exam and notes an irregular adnexal mass and right-sided pleural effusion. The physician decides to send the patient for a transvaginal ultrasound and orders a CA-125 level. Which one of the following facts about the patient most increased her risk for developing this malignancy?
   A. She has given birth to 4 children
   B. She breastfed all her children
   C. Menopause was at 49 for her
   D. Her aunt died of breast cancer at 50
   E. Her age
   F. Her grandmother died of endometrial cancer
   G. She took oral contraceptives for many years when she was not pregnant with her children

2. A 35-year-old G2P0 woman with a clinical history of obesity and hypertension presents to the gynecology clinic with some intermenstrual bleeding. She states that in the past few months her periods have been excessively heavy to the point where she is changing a tampon more often than one every hour and is occasionally passing quarter-sized clots. She also complains of severe pelvic cramping. On bimanual pelvic examination the patient has a slightly enlarged boggy uterus and no adnexal masses or tenderness. The gynecologist asks her to return for endometrial sampling, which

ultimately results in a diagnosis of complex atypical hyperplasia. What is the next most appropriate step in management?

A. Total abdominal hysterectomy
B. Endometrial ablation
C. Progestin therapy
D. Advise the patient to lose weight
E. Repeat endometrial sampling in 3 months
F. Hysteroscopy
G. Dilation and curettage

3. A 17-year-old G0P1 presents to the obstetric clinic complaining of excessive daily vomiting since the beginning of her pregnancy and the sensation that her heart is racing. Her vitals are notable for a blood pressure of 190/100 mm Hg and her uterus is larger than expected for her 16-week pregnancy. On transvaginal ultrasound, her uterus appears to be filled with numerous small hypoechoic vesicles giving a "snowstorm" appearance as well as bilateral multilocular adnexal cysts. Fetal heart sounds cannot be heard. What is this patient's risk for developing malignant sequelae from this pregnancy?

A. 0%
B. 5%
C. 30%
D. 50%
E. 80%

Notes

ANSWERS: What Would Gunner Jess/Jim Do?

1. WWGJD? A 63-year-old woman presents to her primary care doctor with complaints of fatigue, loss of appetite, early satiety, some vague abdominal discomfort, and urinary urgency. She has not been feeling well lately, has been having some difficulty breathing, and thinks she may have even lost some weight. Her physician does a full physical exam as well as a pelvic exam and notes an irregular adnexal mass and right-sided pleural effusion. The physician decides to send the patient for a transvaginal ultrasound and orders a CA-125 level. Which one of the following facts about the patient most increased her risk for developing this malignancy?

Answer: E. Her age

Explanation: The key factors are the patient's age and presenting symptoms. Her symptoms are classic for a gynecologic malignancy: weight loss, early satiety, abdominal discomfort, and urinary urgency, all likely due compression by an enlarging mass, either uterine or ovarian. The patient presents with an irregular adnexal mass, however, and not postmenopausal bleeding, suggesting that ovarian cancer is far more likely than endometrial cancer, which would normally present with some form of AUB. Additionally, description of the uterus is omitted, a pertinent negative, as a uterine malignancy such as leiomyosarcoma or endometrial cancer would likely enlarge the uterus if presenting with bulk symptoms. Pleural effusions are also relatively common presenting signs for serous ovarian adenocarcinoma.

Given the diagnosis of an ovarian malignancy, most of the answer options are actually protective factors against ovarian cancer; multiparity (A), breastfeeding (B), menopause before 52, that is, not late menopause (C), combined oral contraceptives (G). The other answer options are not associated with an increase risk in ovarian cancer—breast cancer or endometrial cancer in a relative that is not a first-degree relative (D, F). Therefore, the only answer left is the correct answer, that her age of 63 increases her risk of developing ovarian cancer (E). Increasing age is a risk factor for epithelial ovarian cancers as the incidence of these cancers increases with age.

2. WWGJD? A 35-year-old G2P0 woman with a clinical history of obesity and hypertension presents to

the gynecology clinic with some **intermenstrual bleeding.** She states that in the past few months her periods have been **excessively heavy** to the point where she is changing a tampon more often than one every hour and is occasionally **passing quarter-sized clots.** She also complains of severe pelvic cramping. On bimanual pelvic examination the patient has a **slightly enlarged boggy uterus** and no adnexal masses or tenderness. The gynecologist asks her to return for endometrial sampling, which ultimately results in a diagnosis of complex atypical hyperplasia. What is the next most appropriate step in management?

Answer: C. Progestin therapy

Explanation: This patient presents with a classic case of endometrial hyperplasia. She has one of the risk factors (obesity) and presents with heavy AUB.

It is important to note that the patient is only 35 years old and may still desire future pregnancy. Therefore, total abdominal hysterectomy (A), which is advised for postmenopausal women with complex atypical hyperplasia, is not a good option for this patient.

Although endometrial ablation (B) would stop the heavy vaginal bleeding, it is absolutely contraindicated in patients who have atypical hyperplasia because it can prevent future endometrial sampling and mask future malignancy.

Although advising the patient to lose weight (D) is a good idea because obesity increases her risk for endometrial cancer, it is not aggressive enough in someone who has atypical hyperplasia with up to a 30% risk of progression to endometrial cancer.

Similarly, simply repeating endometrial sampling in 3 months (E) without any treatment is not aggressive enough.

Hysteroscopy (F) is utilized for direct visualization of the uterine cavity and to guide biopsies of any visible lesions. If endometrial hyperplasia or carcinoma is already found on the initial endometrial sampling, there is no need for hysteroscopy because the patient already warrants treatment.

Finally, D&C (G) is used to remove the contents of the uterine cavity for examination. A D&C would not address the state of unopposed estrogen, and although it would remove some of the hyperplasia, it would not prevent future hyperplasia or carcinoma from developing.

The answer of "progestin therapy" is correct because in this younger woman with the potential desire to continue childbearing, it attempts to treat the hyperplasia without removing the uterus.

3. **WWGJD?** A 17-year-old G0P1 presents to obstetric clinic complaining of excessive **daily vomiting** since the beginning of her pregnancy and the sensation that her **heart is racing.** Her vitals are notable for a blood pressure of 190/100 mm Hg and her **uterus is larger than expected** for her 16-week pregnancy. On transvaginal ultrasound, her uterus appears to be filled with numerous small **hypoechoic vesicles** giving a "snowstorm" **appearance** as well as **bilateral multilocular adnexal cysts.** Fetal heart sounds cannot be heard. What is this patient's risk for developing malignant sequelae from this pregnancy?

Answer: C. 30%

Explanation: This patient is pregnant at a young age, which is a risk factor for a molar pregnancy. She is vomiting excessively (likely as a result of hyperemesis gravidarum, which is often seen in complete molar pregnancies due to the excessively high levels of serum beta-hCG), has preeclampsia (hypertension) prior to 20 weeks, and her uterus is large for gestational age—all signs of a complete molar pregnancy. TVUS reveals a classic appearance of a complete molar pregnancy with no fetal parts and no fetal heart sounds. Also present are bilateral theca lutein cysts (which are also sequelae of high serum beta-hCG). Given how consistent this presentation is with a complete molar pregnancy, the best answer choice is 30% because approximately one-third of all complete molar pregnancies are associated with malignant sequelae. If she had a partial molar pregnancy the risk would be closer to 1%, but not 0%.

Fertility, Infertility, and Birth Control

Kumar Nadhan, Rebecca W. Gao, Hao-Hua Wu, Leo Wang, and Holly W. Cummings

Introduction

Female fertility can be disrupted by hormonal dysregulation, anatomic abnormalities, scarring from prior surgery, and environmental factors such as tobacco use. Some patients seek assistance in preventing pregnancy and others seek assistance in achieving pregnancy.

Contraception

There is an emphasis on providing long-acting, reversible contraceptive devices whenever possible so as to increase contraceptive efficacy. Contraceptives can be hormonal or nonhormonal. Any estrogen-containing contraceptive carries an increased risk of venous thromboembolism, which is often increased in women with additional risk factors, including smoking, obesity, hypertension, and age greater than 35 years.

Table 6.1 describes each contraceptive in further detail.

Sterilization

The most common form of elective sterilization is tubal ligation, colloquially known as "tying the tubes." This is a surgical procedure with irreversible effects, so the decision to undergo sterilization should be carefully discussed.

Buzz Words: Multiple children + happy + husband is aware + does not desire further children

Clinical Presentation: On the exam, the ideal candidate would be a woman >25 with multiple children and a supportive family who has made the decision to not have any more children. She should not be depressed or coerced into this choice.

Prophylaxis (PPx): N/A

Mechanism of Disease (MoD): Laparoscopy → clips or cauterization to block off fallopian tubes

Diagnostic Steps (Dx): N/A

Treatment and Management Steps (Tx/Mgmt):
1. Can be done electively and/or postpartum

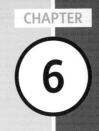

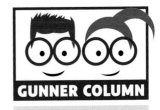

GUNNER COLUMN

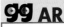
AR
Types of contraception video

TABLE 6.1 Birth Control

Birth Control	Administration	Mechanism of Action	Therapeutic Duration	Benefits	Problems	Efficacy
Tubal ligation	Surgery	Surgical	Permanent	Permanent (best for patients who no longer desire more children)	Possible ectopic pregnancy, cannot be reversed	Extremely high
Nexplanon	Implant in arm	Progestin interferes with ovulation	3 years	Compliance; quick, painless insertion	Scarring around device	Extremely high
IUD (hormonal, copper)	Implant in uterus	(1) Hormonal progestin → interferes with ovulation, cervical mucus (2) Copper → inflammation, obstruction	5 years	Compliance	Copper allergy, inflammation	Extremely high
Ortho Evra	Transdermal patch	Estrogen and progestin interfere with ovulation, (thicken) cervical mucus, and uterine lining	3 weeks	Compliance	Very high blood-clotting risk; deep venous thrombosis, pulmonary embolism	High
Depo-Provera	Intramuscular injection	Progestin	3 months	Compliance	Loss of bone density	High
NuvaRing	Vaginal ring	Estrogen and progestin interfere with ovulation	3 weeks	Noninvasive	May fall out, risk of blood clotting	Moderate-high based on compliance
OCPs	Oral	Estrogen and progestin interfere with ovulation	As long as ingested regularly	Noninvasive	Must be taken daily, risk of blood clotting (DVT/PE)	Moderate-high based on compliance
Mini-pill	Oral	Progestin only interferes with ovulation, (thickens) cervical mucus, cervical lining	As long as ingested regularly	Noninvasive, minimal risk	Must be taken daily on the exact minute	Moderate-high based on compliance
Male condom	Penile cover	Obstruction	Single use	STD protection, cheap	Compliance	Low-high based on compliance
Female diaphragm	Vaginal insertion	Obstruction, spermicidal	Single use	STD protection, female's control	May fall out; must leave in for 6 hours after intercourse	Low
Female condom	Vaginal insertion	Obstruction	Single use	Female's control	Compliance	Low

Female Infertility

Infertility is defined as the inability to become pregnant after 12 months of contraceptive-free regular sexual intercourse. The most common cause of female infertility is ovulatory dysfunction. Although this is not a specific disease process, on the exam you should look for obvious hormone-related diseases like polycystic ovarian syndrome (PCOS) and thyroid dysfunction. The second most common cause of female infertility is tubal obstruction. Other factors that may contribute to infertility include increasing age, smoking, extremes of body weight, and rare pathologies such as Turner syndrome.

Tubal Factor Infertility

Tubal factor infertility (TFI) refers to pathology occurring anywhere in the fallopian tubes. The most common cause of infertility in this category is salpingitis or inflammation of the fallopian tubes, usually from sexually transmitted infections (STIs). Inflammation leads to scarring, which obstructs the passage of the egg through the tubes.

Buzz Words: Young woman + recurrent STIs

Clinical Presentation: A 30-year-old woman with a history of multiple sexual partners without condom usage and several untreated STIs presents with infertility.

PPx: N/A

MoD:
- Hydrosalpinx/pelvic adhesions/fusion of fimbriae → distal tube obstruction
- Infection/endometriosis/myoma → inflammation → proximal tube obstruction

Dx:
1. Hysterosalpingogram (HSG)

Tx/Mgmt:
1. In vitro fertilization (IVF)
2. Tubal reconstruction or removal surgery before IVF if needed

Gonadal Dysgenesis 45, X (Turner Syndrome)

Turner syndrome is a rare chromosomal abnormality in females with the loss of an X chromosome, resulting in a 45X karyotype. The syndrome manifests in a classic constellation of physical features that you may recall from step 1—short stature, shield chest, neck webbing, and lymphedema of the hands and feet. If described in a vignette, consider that the patient may be infertile, as Turner patients often have abnormally developed ovaries ("streak ovaries")

Turner Syndrome

that cause primary amenorrhea or hormonal dysregulation. Note that patients with Turner syndrome can have normal breast and pubic hair development.

Buzz Words: Short + broad chest + neck webbing + primary amenorrhea + no puberty

Clinical Presentation: A 22-year-old woman has not yet had menarche. She is short and has widely spaced nipples as well as additional folds of skin around her neck.

PPx: N/A

MoD: Genetic material from X chromosome lost → abnormal ovary development in embryogenesis → ovarian failure→ primary or secondary amenorrhea

Dx:

1. Clinical presentation
2. definitive diagnosis = karyotype

Tx/Mgmt:

1. Oocyte donation—The reproductive tract besides the ovaries is still intact. Oocyte donation can lead to a viable pregnancy, but the pregnancy will be high-risk.
2. Growth hormone and estrogen for physical development.

GUNNER PRACTICE

1. An 18-year-old patient comes into the outpatient clinic complaining of an inability to conceive. She has been having regular unprotected intercourse with her boyfriend for 11 months. She was on OCPs but discontinued them a year ago. She denies any significant past medical history. Her mother had breast cancer treated with a partial mastectomy. She drinks socially and is a former smoker. She has normal pubic hair distribution but minimal breast development. Menarche was at age 16, but her periods were irregular and stopped completely at age 17. She is short, with wide shoulders, a wide chest, and narrow hips. What is the most likely reason for her infertility?

   A. Has not been enough time since OCP discontinuation
   B. Patient has not been trying for a full 12 months
   C. Nonfunctional endometrium
   D. Nonfunctional gonads
   E. Tobacco and alcohol have made a poor physiologic environment for pregnancy

2. A 20-year-old female desires a form of contraception. She is currently using male condoms intermittently. She doesn't drink alcohol, smokes half a pack of cigarettes

per day, and does not have migraines with aura. She is very afraid of gaining weight on birth control and has a body mass index (BMI) of 21. Her menstrual periods are regular but heavy, requiring five or six pads per day on the heaviest flow day. What is the best form of contraception for this patient?

A. Depo-Provera injection
B. Levonorgestrel IUD
C. Copper IUD
D. Oral contraceptive pills
E. Continuous oral contraceptive pills

ANSWERS: What Would Gunner Jess/Jim Do?

1. WWGJD? An 18-year-old patient comes into the outpatient clinic complaining of an inability to conceive. She has been having regular unprotected intercourse with her boyfriend for 11 months without condoms. She was on OCPs but discontinued them one year ago. She denies any significant past medical history. Her mother had breast cancer treated with a partial mastectomy. She drinks socially and is a former smoker. She has normal pubic hair distribution but minimal breast development. Menarche was at age 16, but her periods were irregular and stopped completely at age 17. She has a short stature with wide shoulders and a wide chest and narrow hips. What is the most likely diagnosis for her infertility?

Answer: D. Nonfunctional gonads

   Explanation: Given the patient's age, lack of menstruation, and physical appearance, she most likely has Turner syndrome. Infertility with Turner syndrome is due to abnormal development of the ovaries, or ovarian dysgenesis. These are nonfunctioning ovaries that often undergo scarring and fibrosis, creating streak ovaries.

   A. Has not been enough time since OCP discontinuation → Incorrect. There is no delay in return to fertility after discontinuing oral contraceptive pills.

   B. Patient has not been trying for a full 12 months → Incorrect. Although this is true, the patient has more concerning reasons for infertility beyond the length of time spent trying.

   C. Nonfunctional endometrium → Incorrect. The endometrium is fully functional in Turner syndrome patients.

   E. Tobacco and alcohol have made a poor physiologic environment for pregnancy → Incorrect. Tobacco and alcohol may contribute to infertility and often delay conception; however, they are not the primary reason for infertility in this patient.

2. WWGJD? A 20-year-old female desires a form of contraception. She is currently using male condoms intermittently. She doesn't drink alcohol, smokes half a pack of cigarettes per day, and does not have migraines with aura. She has no history of DVTs. She is very afraid of gaining weight on birth control and has a BMI of 21. Her menstrual periods are regular but heavy, requiring 5-6 pads/day on the heaviest flow day. What is the best form of contraception for this patient?

Answer: B. Levonorgestrel IUD, a long-acting and effective form of contraception.

A. Depo-Provera injection → Incorrect. There is a risk of weight gain with this method.

C. Copper IUD → Incorrect. The patient has heavy periods, which is a relative contraindication.

D. Oral contraceptive pills → Incorrect. The patient smokes.

E. Continuous oral contraceptive pills → Incorrect. OCP use is contraindicated with tobacco use.

Menopause

Kumar Nadhan, Rebecca W. Gao, Hao-Hua Wu, Leo Wang, and Holly W. Cummings

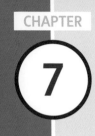

GUNNER COLUMN

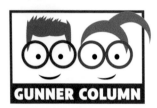

99 AR

ACOG Resource Overview for menopause

Introduction

Menopause is defined as the 12-month period after a female's last menstrual cycle. At this point there are no more functional ovarian follicles and thus no ovulation. The average age of menopause is 51 years, but it can be quite variable. Although the diagnosis can be made clinically, lab values will show **decreased estrogen with increased follicle-stimulating hormone (FSH), luteinizing hormone (LH), and gonadotropin-releasing hormone (GnRH)**. Symptoms such as hot flashes, depression, vaginal atrophy, and lower urinary tract symptoms arise well before menopause owing to declining estrogen levels. This perimenopausal or transitional period may last several years. Low postmenopausal estrogen increases the risk of osteoporosis and heart disease. For your exam, you must know the normal presentation of menopause as well as abnormal presentation time and symptoms. All the conditions presented here are related to the process of menopause and its correlating hormonal changes.

Menopause

Buzz Words: Atrophic, friable vaginal mucosa + scant blood in vaginal canal + small blood stains on underwear past 6 months + dyspareunia + normal uterus + last menses at least 12 months earlier

Clinical Presentation: Patients are often above age 45 years without menses but with hot flashes and sleep disturbances for at least 12 months. Smokers may have an earlier onset of menopause.

Prophylaxis (PPx): There are no prophylactic measures to prevent menopause. However, menopausal women require prophylaxis against other disorders, such as calcium for osteoporosis.

Mechanism of Disease (MoD): No more ovarian follicles → ovaries no longer making estrogen → hypoestrogenic state. Once menopause hits, aromatase in ovaries ceases to work, and the small amount of aromatase in peripheral tissues take over to convert adrenal androgens to estrogens. Adipose tissue contains aromatase, so obese patients may have less severe symptoms of menopause.

Diagnostic Steps (Dx):

1. Pelvic exam
2. Thyroid-stimulating hormone (TSH) and FSH to rule out other pathology, like hyperthyroidism
3. Urinalysis and urine culture

Treatment and Management Steps (Tx/Mgmt):

1. Vaginal estrogen replacement
2. Hormone replacement therapy (estrogen + progestin) (HRT):
   - Contraindicated in patients with vaginal bleeding; must r/o cancer first
   - HRT most effective treatment for hot flashes + night sweats + vaginal dryness
   - Slight risk in breast cancer + cardiovascular disease (CVD), myocardial infarction (MI), stroke, thrombo-embolic events
   - **Increases high-density lipoprotein (HDL) and decreases low-density lipoprotein (LDL),** since estrogen increases triglycerides, LDL catabolism, and lipoprotein receptor numbers. Estrogen also inhibits **hepatic lipase activity,** which prevents conversion of HDL2 to HDL3 (to increase HDL levels).
   - Calcium replacement

Premature Menopause/Primary Ovarian Insufficiency

Buzz Words: Thirties + irregular menses + menopausal symptoms + elevated FSH

Clinical Presentation: A 35-year-old female presents with irregular menstrual cycles, oligomenorrhea, or amenorrhea. May have a history of ovarian damage via surgery, chemo, or radiation. Tobacco use is also associated with premature ovarian failure.

PPx: N/A

MoD: Hypothalamic-pituitary-ovarian axis dysfunction, creating a false menopause

Dx:

1. Elevated FSH at postmenopausal levels
2. Serum hCG to rule out pregnancy

Tx/Management:

1. Manage as a postmenopausal woman—treat symptomatically and address increased risk of osteoporosis and cardiovascular disease.

Perimenopause

Buzz Words: Late 40s + irregular cycles + hot flashes + sleep disturbance + mood changes

Clinical Presentation: The years leading up to menopause, when amount of estrogen produced starts to vary widely, which is manifested by the start of irregular cycles.

PPx: N/A

MoD: Fluctuating estrogen levels

Dx:

1. Clinical presentation.
2. Confirmed with high FSH and estradiol, but may appear normal as levels will be fluctuating.

Tx/Management:

1. Same as for menopause: symptomatic management and/or HRT.

Premenopausal Menorrhagia

Buzz Words: Forties + unpredictable with no history of heavy menses + oligomenorrhea

Clinical Presentation: A 43-year-old woman with previously normal menstrual cycles has unsually heavy periods spaced further apart than usual.

PPx: N/A

MoD: Oligomenorrhea → anovulation → unopposed estrogen → endometrial proliferation longer than one cycle → endometrium outgrows blood supply → sloughing throughout cycle or buildup to end of cycle

Dx:

1. Rule out pregnancy

Tx/Management:

1. Nonsteroidal anti-inflammatory drugs (NSAIDs) → reduce prostaglandins → reduce blood flow
2. Discuss hormone replacement therapy for menopause

Postmenopausal Atrophic Vaginitis/ Vaginal Atrophy

Buzz Words: Postmenopausal + dyspareunia + lower urinary symptoms+ pale, dry, smooth vaginal epithelium + scarce pubic hair + loss of labial fat pad + **dysuria** + vaginal dryness

Clinical Presentation: A postmenopausal woman presents with dysuria, vaginal dryness, and pain with sexual intercourse.

PPx: N/A

MoD: Decreased estrogen → disruption of vaginal and urinary tract epithelium → thinning, dryness, inflammation → epithelial cell death

Dx:
1. Clinical presentation

Tx/Mgmt
1. Vaginal lubricant
2. Estrogen cream for vaginal use

Postmenopausal Bleeding

Any bleeding, even minimal, is abnormal after menopause and should be concerning.

Clinical Presentation: A postmenopausal woman (age 50+) presents with vaginal bleeding.

PPx: N/A

MoD:
- Endometrial atrophy—80% of cases
- Endometrial cancer—15% of cases
- Endometrial polyp

Dx: N/A

Tx/Mgmt:
Rule out cancer → endometrial biopsy or dilation and curettage (D&C)

Vasomotor Symptoms

Buzz Words: Perimenopausal + night sweats + anxiety + blushing

Clinical Presentation: Hot flashes are the most common manifestation of menopause.

PPx: Estrogen therapy

MoD: Declining estrogen → hypothalamic dysfunction → inappropriate vasodilation

Dx:
1. Clinical presentation

Tx/Mgmt:
1. Behavioral (maintaining lower body temperature—light clothing, fans, etc.)
2. HRT

QUICK TIPS
Hormone (estrogen and progesterone) therapy (HRT)
   Indications: Osteoporosis Prophylaxis, Hot Flashes, Urogenital Atrophy, Vasomotor Symptoms
   Contraindications: Thromboembolic Disease, Breast/Endometrial Cancer, Endometriosis

GUNNER PRACTICE

1. A 49-year-old woman comes to your office complaining of multiple 2-minute episodes over the last 6 months of intense heat over her chest and face. She hasn't taken any medication during the episodes but feels better when she places a cold compress on her forehead. She is anxious because she cannot predict when they will occur. Ten months earlier she traveled to the Sahara for 3 weeks and is worried she has a bug like Zika. What is the appropriate first step in managing this patient's symptoms?

A. Reassurance
B. Estrogen
C. Behavior modification
D. Urgent admission and quarantine
E. Hormonal replacement therapy

2. A 31-year-old woman has had irregular periods for the last 2 years, involving months without menses and then months with heavy bleeding. She has a history of radiation for an abdominal cancerous lymph node. She has a healthy 6-year-old girl but wants one more child. What is the patient's best option for having an additional child?

A. Clomiphene
B. Estrogen therapy
C. Estrogen and progesterone therapy
D. In vitro fertilization
E. Basal temperature measurement

Notes

ANSWERS: What Would Gunner Jess/Jim Do?

1. WWGJD? A 49-year-old woman comes to your office complaining of multiple 2-minute episodes over the last 6 months of intense heat over her chest and face. She hasn't taken any medication during the episodes, but she feels better when she places a cold compress on her forehead. She is anxious because she cannot predict when they will occur. Ten months ago, she traveled to the Sahara for 3 weeks and is worried she has a bug like Zika. What is the appropriate first step in management of this patient's symptoms?

Answer: C. Behavior modification

Explanation: The patient is experiencing perimenopausal vasomotor symptoms or hot flashes. She is about the age when you would expect her to enter menopause. Behavior modification like light clothing and room temperature control should be attempted before HRT.

A. Reassurance → Incorrect. Hot flashes are a clear sign of perimenopause and the patient should be informed of further changes that may occur in her body.

B. Estrogen → Incorrect. HRT is a first-line therapy for perimenopausal symptoms. Hot flashes in particular are a leading indication for estrogen therapy; however, the patient has a thromboembolic history, which is a contraindication for hormone therapy.

D. Urgent admission and quarantine → Incorrect. The presentation is classic of hot flashes rather than an exotic bug like Zika. Hot flashes are a common presentation of perimenopause and do not require hospital admission. They can be easily treated in the outpatient clinic.

E. Hormonal replacement therapy → Incorrect. Although the patient is experiencing hot flashes and appears to have menopause, remember that the first step is to modify behavior.

2. WWGJD? A 31-year-old woman has had irregular periods for the last 2 years, involving months without menses and then months with heavy bleeding. She has a history of radiation for an abdominal cancerous lymph node. She has one healthy 6-year-old girl, but wants one more child. What is the patient's best option for having an additional child?

Answer: D. In vitro fertilization

Explanation: The patient is experience premature ovarian insufficiency (POI) or premature menopause. As in menopause, the ovaries are no longer functional in POI. However, she has had a successful previous pregnancy, which means that her endometrium is viable. Therefore IVF is the most viable option.

A. Clomiphene → Incorrect. Clomiphene may be used for infertility, as it stimulates ovulation in anovulatory patients. However, patients with POI no longer have functional ovarian follicles to be stimulated.

B. Estrogen therapy → Incorrect. Estrogen levels may help diagnose POI, but that is not a treatment for infertility.

C. Estrogen and progesterone therapy → Incorrect. Hormone therapy is not a treatment for infertility.

E. Basal temperature measurement → Incorrect. It is almost never correct to ask patient's to monitor only basal temperature in order to conceive.

Menstrual and Endocrine Disorders

Hao-Hua Wu, Leo Wang, Rebecca W. Gao, and Holly W. Cummings

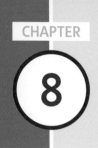

Introduction

This chapter is one of the highest yielding on the Ob/Gyn Shelf. It revolves around understanding the differential of four chief complaints: (1) meno- or metrorrhagia, (2) amenorrhea, (3) dysmenorrhea, and (4) pelvic pain. Although there is no official National Board of Medical Examiners (NBME) breakdown, it is likely that you will see at least 15 questions on your shelf related to those four chief complaints.

It is critical to do questions related to abnormal bleeding (e.g., abnormal uterine bleeding [AUB], amenorrhea) early, so start early with Gunner Practice, UWorld, or uWise. Do not get discouraged if you don't understand or memorize the material of this chapter on your first pass. You will likely need to peruse and apply this material multiple times before being ready for the exam. Thus, plan accordingly with your study schedule.

This chapter is organized into (1) Normal Bleeding and the Hypothalamic-Pituitary-Ovarian (HPO) Axis, (2) Abnormal Bleeding, (3) Abnormal Discomfort, and (4) Gunner Practice.

Normal Bleeding and the Hypothalamic-Pituitary-Ovarian Axis

Patients of reproductive age (12–50 y/o on the shelf) expect to have normal bleeding according to their menstrual cycle. Although normal bleeding will not be directly tested on the shelf, know the following facts to distinguish normal from abnormal bleeding:

Normal Bleeding

- **Average menstrual cycle**: 28 ± 7 days
- **Length of bleeding during menstrual period**: 5 days
- **Volume of blood**: <80 mL for the entire menses
- **Timing of ovulation**: 14 days before menstrual period
- **Mechanism of normal bleeding (HPO axis):**
  Gonadotropin-releasing hormone (GnRH) from hypothalamus stimulates luteinizing hormone/follicle-stimulating hormone (LH/FSH) from the anterior pituitary → LH/FSH stimulate ovarian follicles to produce estrogen and

progesterone → estrogen builds up the lining of the endometrium, progesterone keeps the endometrial lining from sloughing off → menses when there is a sudden decrease in level of progesterone

Types of Abnormal Bleeding

- **Menorrhagia**: Heavier bleeding than usual either by length (longer than 5 days) or by volume (filling a pad in less than 1 hour)
- **Metrorrhagia**: Bleeding in between cycles—for example, a woman with 35-day cycles bleeds at day 14
- **Menometrorrhagia**: Heavier bleeding **and** bleeding that occurs in between cycles
- **Amenorrhea**: No bleeding when bleeding is expected

Abnormal Bleeding

Abnormal bleeding refers to the unexpected presence or absence of blood during the menstrual cycle in a reproductive-age female (age 12–50 years). Meno-, metro-, and menometrorrhagia as well as amenorrhea are all considered types of "abnormal bleeding" by the NBME.

This section is incredibly high-yield. You will get at least 10 questions where the patient's chief complaint is either unexpected bleeding or unexpected lack of bleeding (primary or secondary amenorrhea). To answer these questions, understand the differential diagnosis for each chief complaint, keep a keen eye for buzz words, learn the appropriate diagnostic tests for a given age group, and know at least one treatment modality for each disorder.

It is very hard to memorize this subsection on your first pass. Be sure to reference these topics multiple times over the course of study. Also, many of the etiologies for abnormal bleeding—including neoplasms, congenital disorders, and medication side effects—are covered in greater detail in other chapters. Make sure you flip between the pages to synthesize learning across several topics.

Differential Diagnosis for Meno-, Metro-, and Menometrorrhagia on the Shelf

Use the following DDx outline to give you the big picture of what to look for when the chief complaint is bleeding from the vagina. A good way to group the differential is by age: prepubertal, reproductive, and menopausal.

Prepubertal age (<12 years) is the age before females begin menses. For the shelf, the most common causes of abnormal bleeding are:

> **QUICK TIP**
>
> Abnormal bleeding ≠ Abnormal uterine bleeding; the latter is a subcategory of the former

APGO abnormal bleeding video

- Foreign body (e.g., toys or toilet paper)
- Sexual abuse (r/o with history and physical exam)
- Pituitary adenomas/craniopharyngiomas
- Congenital disorders

Work up with a pelvic exam, speculum under anesthesia if too painful, computed tomography/magnetic resonance imaging (CT/MRI) to r/o neoplasms, and karyotype analysis to rule out genetic disorders.

Reproductive age (12–50 years) is the age when the menstrual cycle has normalized and ovulation is occurring at regular intervals. These patients typically present with abnormal uterine bleeding (AUB) despite having had a history regular menstrual cycles. Exceptions to the regularity of menstrual cycles occur in young reproductive (ages 12–16) and perimenopausal (ages 45–50) females. These patients may report AUB due to irregularity in ovulation; pubertal females may have irregular ovulation due to lack of ovarian maturity; and perimenopausal females may have irregular ovulation due to depletion of oocytes.

By far the most important cause of AUB in reproductive-age females is pregnancy (regular or ectopic). Any reproductive-age female requires a urine pregnancy test as the first step of workup. Other than that, make sure to rule out the PALM-COEIN (Fig. 8.1) causes of AUB for this age group, as follows:

1. Pap smear to r/o malignancy
2. Wet prep to r/o infections such as bacterial vaginosis, gonorrhea
3. Transvaginal ultrasound to r/o structural abnormalities (e.g., polyps, fibroids, adenomyosis)
4. Dilation and curettage to evaluate the endometrium
5. Hysteroscopy for definitive view and biopsy of the endometrium

QUICK TIP

For prepubertal-age patients who are septic, be on the lookout for **toxic shock syndrome**, which can occur because of a vaginal foreign body.

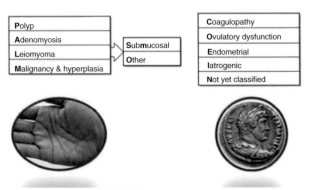

Polyp			Coagulopathy
Adenomyosis		Submucosal	Ovulatory dysfunction
Leiomyoma		Other	Endometrial
Malignancy & hyperplasia			Iatrogenic
			Not yet classified

FIG. 8.1 PALM-COEIN mnemonic created by FIGO.

Although principles of treatment vary widely, remember that the shelf favors the use of contraception (e.g., barrier or hormonal) and that iron supplementation (for the Fe-anemia that occurs owing to blood loss) is usually a good idea.

Menopausal age (>50 years) is the age when females have depleted their oocyte reserves and their ovaries no longer produce estrogen. The most common causes of abnormal bleeding are atrophy of the vagina, cervix, and the endometrium as well as bleeding from hormone replacement therapy (HRT). The most concerning cause of bleeding on the shelf is carcinoma (see Chapter 5). **Workup for this age group must always first exclude neoplasms** through Pap smear or biopsy of the cervix and endometrium. Treatment depends on etiology, but a commonly tested concept is the need for lubrication to prevent postcoital bleeding (less estrogen, less natural vaginal lubrication).

Abnormal Uterine Bleeding (Dysfunctional Uterine Bleeding)

Buzz Words: Uterine bleeding + bleeding longer/heavier than usual (menorrhaghia) + bleeding at abnormal intervals (metrorrhagia)

Clinical Presentation: AUB is menstrual bleeding from the uterus that occurs longer than usual or at irregular intervals. It is important to know the buzz words of the specific disorders that cause AUB, such as polyps, leiomyomas, or neoplasms.

Causes of AUB are classically organized into the mnemonic PALM-COEIN:

- Polyps
- Adenomyosis
- Leiomyoma (submucosal vs. other)
- Malignancy and hyperplasia
- Coagulopathy
- Ovulatory dysfunction
- Endometrial
- Iatrogenic
- Not yet classified

You do NOT have to memorize this mnemonic to do well on the shelf. PALM-COEIN is meant to serve as a broad overview of etiologies of AUB that can be present in a reproductive female. It is more high-yield to memorize the buzz words and workup of the individual disorders, such as adenomyosis or leiomyoma.

The PALM causes are all physical structures that cause AUB, and they are the most high-yield AUB topics on

99 FOR THE WARDS/AR

You may encounter diagnoses such as AUB-O, AUB-A, etc. The letter attached after the hyphen is the letter indicating the PALM-COEIN etiology of bleed (e.g. AUB-O means AUB due to ovulatory dysfunction). This is not tested on the shelf but may be asked by your resident or attending.

the shelf. These causes can be organized by the shape and size of the uterus:

- **Polyps.** Outgrowths within the endometrial cavity that do not enlarge the uterus
- **Adenomyosis.** Symmetrically enlarged uterus due to growth of endometrial glands within the myometrium
- **Leiomyoma** (aka fibroids). Asymmetrically enlarged uterus due to random growths
- **Malignancy and hyperplasia of the endometrium.** Can present as asymmetric growths

The COEIN causes are all nonstructural, and include:

- **Coagulopathies.** May occur if patient has a bleeding diathesis and vessels cannot clot fast enough
- **Ovulatory dysfunction.** Early pubertal (11–15 years) or perimenopausal (48–51 years) age groups when ovulation is either just starting to occur or occurs less and less frequently
- **Endometrial.** Causes such as insufficient production of local vasoconstrictors (e.g., prostaglandin F2) OR infection of the endometrium due to sexually transmitted disease
- **Iatrogenic.** From medication (e.g., breakthrough bleeding from hormonal therapy, concomitant use of blood thinners)
- **Not yet classified.** Not very well defined, such as arteriovenous malformation (This is not frequently tested.)

Prophylaxis (PPx):

- Avoid blood thinners such as warfarin, heparin
- Contraception to avoid sexually transmitted infections (STIs)

Mechanism of Disease (MoD): The mechanism is determined by the cause of bleeding. The most important mechanism to know is bleeding due to ovulatory dysfunction, also known as periods of abnormal anovulation. For example, if there is unopposed estrogen stimulation of the endometrium but no progesterone being made (either from failure of corpus luteum development or gaps in oral contraceptive use), then the patient can experience unexpected, noncyclic bleeding. Bleeding due to ovulatory dysfunction is most commonly seen in patients at the beginning of puberty or in perimenopausal women. In puberty, ovulation is not occurring regularly due to immaturity of the HPA axis. In perimenopause, ovulation is not occurring regularly due to the depletion of oocytes.

99 AR

High yield vaginal bleeding video

Diagnostic Steps (Dx):

1. Laboratory tests to include:
   - Complete blood count (CBC)
   - Beta-hCG to r/o pregnancy (AUB cannot be diagnosed in pregnant patient)
   - Coags (PT, PTT, aPTT, fibrinogen)
   - Ristocetin cofactor assay and von Willebrand factor (vWF) factor antigen to r/o vWF
   - Thyroid-stimulating hormone (TSH)
   - Iron, total-iron binding capacity (TIBC), ferritin
2. Transvaginal ultrasound to r/o structural pathology
3. Additional age-related workup:
   - If 13–39 y/o → LH, FSH, and androgen testing to r/o polycystic ovarian syndrome (PCOS)
   - If ≥40 y/o, endometrial biopsy to r/o neoplasm
4. Hysteroscopy or saline infusion sonohysterography in patients who have failed medical management

Treatment and Management Steps (Tx/Mgmt):

1. For AUB due to ovulatory dysfunction:
   - Progestins
   - Levonorgestrel IUD
   - Hysterectomy w/o cervical preservation for women who do not want to have children
2. For AUB due to structural causes (e.g., PALM):
   - Surgical removal of polyp or fibroid
   - Hysterectomy for adenomyosis, malignancy

Endometrial Polyp

Buzz Words: AUB + single mass in uterus on ultrasound + no uterine enlargement → endometrial polyp

Clinical Presentation: Endometrial polyps are masses that grow from the endometrial tissue within the uterus; they can lead to abnormal bleeding due to thin blood vessels that supply the polyp. Polyps are mostly benign but there is a small risk of neoplasm. Because of this small risk, polypectomy is often the definitive treatment.

PPx: N/A

MoD: Unknown

Dx:

1. Pelvic exam
2. Beta-hCG
3. Transvaginal ultrasound
4. Hysteroscopy

Tx/Mgmt:

1. Polypectomy (hysteroscopic resection) to relieve symptoms and reduce risk of malignant transformation

QUICK TIP

W/u different according to age. PCOS common in young females and neoplastic risk higher in perimenopausal females.

QUICK TIP

Avoid endometrial ablation in young females. Can compromise accuracy of future endometrial biopsy.

99 FOR THE WARDS

Epidemiology of polyps as cancerous and precancerous lesions

99 AR

Systematic review of treatment of endometrial polyps

Adenomyosis

Buzz Words: Dysmenorrhea + pelvic pain + AUB (menor-rhagia) + bulky, globular, tender, **boggy** uterus + multiparous + >40 y/o **+ symmetrically enlarged uterus**

Clinical Presentation: Adenomyosis exists when ectopic glandular tissue is found in the myometrium of the uterus. Over 50% of patients with adenomyosis have a concurrent fibroid. Patients present with an enlarged, symmetric uterus, and adenomyosis is on the differential for both AUB and dysmenorrhea.

PPx: N/A

MoD: Endometrial glands invade uterine musculature → blood deposits between smooth muscle fibers of myometrium → ectopic endometrium bleeds

- Uterus gradually increases in size due to accumulation of the deposited blood

Dx:
1. Ultrasound
2. If >45 y/o with irregular menstrual bleeding → endometrial biopsy to r/o malignancy
3. **Hysterectomy** + surgical pathology = definitive diagnosis

Tx/Mgmt:
1. Nonsteroidal anti-inflammatory drugs (NSAIDs)
2. Oral contraceptive pills (OCPs) or progestins
3. Danazol or continuous GnRH (mimicking menopause would lead to a decrease in adenomyosis)
4. Endometrial ablation
5. Hysterectomy

Leiomyomata Uteri ("Fibroids," Uterine Leiomyomas)

Buzz Words: Enlarged uterus + irregular + mobile uterus with posterior mass + **chronic constipation** + lower abdominal discomfort + >30 y/o + **urinary frequency** + difficulty with pregnancy + **heavy, prolonged menstrual bleeding** with normal cycles

Patient Presentation: Fibroids are diagnosed in reproductive-age women, with a higher incidence in Black women. **See Chapter 5 for full description.**

Amenorrhea

Amenorrhea is the absence of bleeding from menses when bleeding is expected. It is divided into primary and secondary amenorrhea.

QUICK TIP

Most noteworthy symptom in fibroids is menorrhagia.

- **Primary amenorrhea**: Absence of menstrual bleeding by 16 years of age + no previous menses
- **Secondary amenorrhea**: Previously had menses + absence of menstrual bleeding ≥3 months if regular cycles or ≥6 months if irregular cycles

This subsection provides the algorithm for how to diagnose causes of primary and secondary amenorrhea, although some disorders, such as Kallmann syndrome, are covered in more detail in other chapters.

Primary Amenorrhea

Buzz Words: ≥16 y/o girl + never had menses

Clinical Presentation: Primary amenorrhea is the absence of menstrual bleeding by 16 years of age. It can be caused by a lack of hormones (LH, FSH, steroids), dysfunction of end-organ receptors, or outflow tract obstruction.

Instead of memorizing these etiologies all at once, refer back to this page as you begin to learn the Buzz Words, Dx, and Tx/Mgmt of these disorders in other chapters. Most of the disorders have such distinct Buzz Words (e.g., *anosmia* for Kallman syndrome, *hairless individual* for androgen insensitivity syndrome) that you can ascertain the diagnosis on the shelf without having to know that the patient has associated primary amenorrhea. The purpose of this subsection is to give you a general overview of causes of primary amenorrhea that are high-yield for the shelf.

PPx: N/A

MoD: Three things can prevent the appearance of menstrual bleeding before the age of 16:

- Problem with hormone production (decreased LH/FSH):
  - Mechanism: Insufficient production of central hormones (GnRH, LH, FSH) or sex steroids (testosterone)
  - Examples:
    - Pituitary adenoma or craniopharyngioma: Pituitary compression, loss of peripheral vision
    - Kallman syndrome: Lack of hypothalamic nuclei to produce GnRH, anosmia
    - 17-alpha-hydoxylase deficiency: 46XY, no testosterone production, hypertension
    - Hypogonadotrophic hypogonadism: Stress due to excessive exercise or eating disorder increases cortisol → cortisol inhibits GnRH → amenorrhea

99 AR

Premature ovarian failure video

QUICK TIP

Hypogonadotrophic hypogonadism can also be secondary amenorrhea.

- Problem with end-organ response to hormone (increased LH/FSH):
  - Mechanism: End reproductive organ (ovaries) unable to respond central hormones or sex steroids
  - Examples:
    - Turner syndrome: XO, streak ovaries
    - XY gonadal dysgenesis (Swyer syndrome): 46 XY, no SRY, streak gonads
    - Androgen insensitivity syndrome: 46XY, no testosterone receptor, blind-pouch vagina, no virilization
- Problem with outflow tract (normal LH/FSH):
  - Mechanism: Problem with outflow tract (uterus to opening of vaginal canal) that prevents blood flow
  - Examples:
    - Imperforate hymen: Menses occurring but blood cannot get out due to hymenal obstruction, **hematocolpos**
    - Vaginal atresia: Distal vaginal canal fails to form, replaced by fibrotic tissue
    - Transverse septum: Abnormal formation of septum due to improper fusion of Mullerian duct to urogenital sinus
    - **Müllerian agenesis** (aka Mayer–Rokitansky–Kuster–Hauser syndrome): 46 XX, no uterus, external genitalia present, virilization

Dx:
1. Pelvic ultrasound to r/o outflow tract obstruction
2. LH/FSH levels
3. Karyotype analysis (if FSH increased)
4. Cranial MRI (if FSH decreased)
5. Testosterone levels (if uterus absent)
6. 17-hydroxyprogesterone to r/o congenital adrenal hyperplasia

Tx/Mgmt:
1. Depends on etiology (covered in more detail in other chapters):
   - Pituitary adenoma or craniopharyngioma → hormone replacement + resection of tumor
   - 17-alpha-hydroxylase deficiency → hormone replacement
   - Hypogonadotrophic hypogonadism → decrease stress/exercise intensity + treatment of eating disorder (e.g., anorexia or bulimia) + **pulsatile** GnRH release
   - Kallman syndrome → hormone replacement
   - Turner syndrome → hormone replacement
   - Androgen insensitivity syndrome and Swyer syndrome → removal of gonadal structures

99 AR

Video of primary amenorrhea etiology

QUICK TIPS

GnRH deficiency cannot be treated with continuous GnRH release because of receptor desensitization; pulsatile is the best approach.

QUICK TIPS

If Y chromosome is present, bilateral oophorectomy is recommended to ppx ovarian germ cell neoplasm.

Outflow tract disorders (i.e., imperforate hymen, vaginal atresia, transverse septum) → surgery to open up outflow tract

Secondary Amenorrhea

Buzz Words:
- History of regular menstrual cycles + reproductive age female + amenorrhea for 3 months
- History of irregular menstrual cycles + amenorrhea for 6 months

Clinical Presentation: A 30 y/o female with regular periods presents with amenorrhea for 3 months.

PPx: (1) Avoidance of excessive exercise and manage eating disorders. (2) OCPs

MoD: The etiology of secondary amenorrhea can be divided into three categories:
- **Pregnancy** (regular or ectopic): Most common cause, progesterone produced by corpus luteum prevents endometrial lining from shedding
- **Exogenous:** Side effect of medications and drugs. Most high-yield for Ob/Gyn shelf are antipsychotics, which are dopamine antagonists. No dopamine → no prolactin inhibition → too much prolactin → prolactin shuts down HPO axis.
- **HPO axis abnormality:**
  - Hypothalamic dysfunction
  - Hypogonadotrophic hypogonadism (functional hypothalamic amenorrhea)
  - Anterior pituitary dysfunction
  - Hypothyroidism (low T3/T4 → no TRH inhibition/ high TRH levels → TRH inhibition of anterior pituitary)
  - Sheehan syndrome (pituitary ischemia s/p postpartum hemorrhage)
  - Pituitary apoplexy (pituitary hemorrhage)
  - Prolactinoma
  - Hyperprolactinemia (overproduction due to decreased dopamine or increased pituitary stimulation)
  - Ovarian dysfunction
  - Gonadotrophin-resistant ovary syndrome (Savage syndrome): Ovary unresponsive to LH/FSH due to defect in receptors
  - PCOS
  - Premature ovarian failure
  - Menopause
  - Endometrial/cervical dysfunction
  - Asherman syndrome
  - Cervical stenosis

99 AR
HPO axis explained

QUICK TIPS
Premature ovarian failure = loss of ovarian function ≤40 y/o

99 FOR THE WARDS

Details of progesterone withdrawal test

Dx:
1. Urine pregnancy test
2. Progesterone withdrawal challenge test to r/o PCOS
3. Estrogen and progesterone test to r/o Asherman
4. LH/FSH to r/o pituitary pathology
5. TSH, T3/T4 to r/o hypothyroidism
6. TVUS
7. Head MRI to r/o pituitary pathology/neoplasm

Tx/Mgmt:
1. Dependent on etiology:
- Hypogonadotrophic hypogonadism → decrease stress/exercise intensity + treatment of eating disorder (e.g., anorexia or bulimia) + **pulsatile** GnRH release
- Hypothyroidism → thyroid hormone
- Sheehan → hormone replacement
- Hyperprolactinemia/prolactinoma → bromocriptine (dopamine agonist that downregulates prolactin)
- PCOS → clomiphene (if patient desires pregnancy), OCPs, treatment of hypertension and diabetes
- Savage syndrome → HRT
- Asherman syndrome → hysteroscopy and estrogen therapy
- Cervical stenosis → surgery

Polycystic Ovarian Syndrome (PCOS, Stein–Leventhal Syndrome)

99 AR

PCOS video

Buzz Words: Hirsutism + acne + male-pattern baldness + amenorrhea/oligorrhea + multiple cysts in ovaries + acanthosis

Clinical Presentation: PCOS is a common cause of secondary amenorrhea. It is diagnosed if patients meet two of three Rotterdam criteria: (1) laboratory or clinical signs (e.g., male-pattern baldness, acne, or hirsutism) of high serum androgen present, (2) amenorrhea or oligomenorrhea, (3) cystic ovaries seen on pelvic ultrasound. Because insulin resistance is a characteristic of PCOS, patients are at increased risk of diabetes, dyslipidemia, cardiovascular disease, and metabolic syndrome. In addition, patients have increased risk of endometrial hyperplasia and endometrial cancer due to unopposed estrogen from anovulatory cycles.

PPx: None to prevent PCOS: Once patient has PCOS, ppx diabetes and cardiovascular disease

MoD: Unknown but associated with insulin resistance, cystic ovaries, and hyperandrogenism

Dx:
1. Clinical evaluation (Rotterdam criteria)
2. Pelvic ultrasound of ovaries
3. Testosterone levels (elevated)

4. FSH/LH (elevated, LH > FSH, higher LH:FSH ratios)
5. Glucose tolerance test (>140 two-hour GTT → insulin resistance; >200 two-hour GTT → diabetes mellitus)
6. Fasting lipid panel for all newly diagnosed patients

Tx/Mgmt:
1. Metformin:
   - Prevents T2DM, helps lose weight
   - Helps induce ovulation in PCOS (mechanism unknown but likely by altering insulin levels to allow for more favorable ovulation)
   - Suppresses androgen production by decreasing ovarian gluconeogenesis (helps correct hirsutism)
2. Lifestyle/diet to control diabetes/weight
3. Clomiphene citrate:
   - Addition of estrogen analog improves GnRH/FSH release; used to induce ovulation for patients seeking fertility
4. Ketoconazole
5. Spironolactone

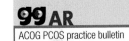

ACOG PCOS practice bulletin

Abnormal Discomfort

Dysmenorrhea

Pain during menses; can be either primary or secondary. Causes of secondary dysmenorrhea, such as adenomyosis and fibroids, frequently overlap with causes of AUB.

Primary Dysmenorrhea

Buzz Words:
- Suprapubic, pelvic pain + nausea and vomiting just before or during menses + normal pelvic exam + teenager (soon after onset of menarche) + regular menses + no risk of STI
- Normal pelvic exam + crampy lower abdomen/back pain during menses + young girl

Clinical Presentation: Primary dysmenorrhea is cramping before or during menstruation without concomitant disease pathology. Patients are usually <25 y/o and do not exhibit other systemic findings as in premenstrual disorder (e.g., breast tenderness or abdominal bloating). The pain of primary dysmenorrhea is greatest on day 2 of menses, when the flow is heaviest. If the patient is >25 y/o and complains of dysmenorrhea, suspect other pathology.

PPx: NSAIDs before the start of menses

MoD: During endometrial sloughing, the disintegrating endometrial cells release prostaglandin F2 alpha as menstruation begins → increased uterine tone → stronger more frequent uterine contractions

Dx:
1. Clinical history to r/o secondary amenorrhea
2. Pelvic exam
3. Test for STIs

Tx/Mgmt:
1. NSAIDs (downregulate prostaglandins through the inhibition of prostaglandin synthetase)
2. OCPs
3. Medroxyprogesterone PO (a type of progestin) is second-line from OCPs (because it doesn't prevent pregnancy)
4. Combination of OCP and NSAIDs in refractory cases

Premenstrual Syndrome

Buzz Words:
- Mood swings + irritability + bloating + breast tenderness + fatigue + decreased libido + anxiety + difficulty concentrating + occur 1–2 weeks prior to menses + resolve with onset of menstrual flow → premenstrual syndrome (PMS)
- Very prominent irritability + very prominent anger + PMS-like symptoms → premenstrual dysphoric disorder

Clinical Presentation: PMS is the constellation of symptoms that occur in the time leading up to and during a woman's menstrual period. On the shelf, this disorder is frequently confused with primary dysmenorrhea, as both present as pain during menses. However, patients with PMS will also report breast tenderness and psychological symptoms such as mood swings, irritability, and anxiety. Patients with PMS will always present with significant disruption of work or activities of daily living, whereas patients with normal menses will be able to carry on their daily activities normally.

Patients with PMS who demonstrate prominent anger and extreme irritability may have **premenstrual dysphoric disorder (PMDD)**. PMDD is a psychiatric diagnosis in DSM-V and can be recognized on the shelf as patients with lability of mood, anger, anxiety, and depression for the majority of menstrual cycles.

PPx: Reduction of caffeine and alcohol intake
MoD: Unknown
Dx:
1. Keep a menstrual diary for 2–3 months

Tx/Mgmt:
1. If PMS → NSAIDs for pain, OCPs to reduce mood fluctuation
2. If PMDD → selective serotonin reuptake inhibitors (SSRIs)

Secondary Dysmenorrhea

Secondary dysmenorrhea is pain during menses caused by concomitant medical pathology such as endometriosis, adenomyosis, fibroids, or adhesions from surgical trauma. The most high-yield of these is endometriosis, which can also appear on the Medicine shelf. Other etiologies of secondary dysmenorrhea, such as adenomyosis and fibroids, were covered earlier.

Endometriosis

Buzz Words:
- **Chronic pelvic pain** (worsens before menses) + dyspareunia + dysmenorrhea for 2 years + regular menses + nodularity over uterosacral area + 27 y/o with retroverted uterus + tender adnexa that are normal in size
- Thickening of uterosacral ligaments + decreased uterine mobility + **infertility** + **homogenous cystic-appearing mass** in left ovary

Clinical Presentation: Endometriosis is the appearance of endometrial tissue outside the uterus, causing pelvic pain. Ectopic endometrial tissue can implant in a variety of places, including the ovaries, appendix, sigmoid colon, round ligament, and broad ligaments. Almost 50% of patients with endometriosis are infertile.

A common cause of secondary dysmenorrhea. Exam will show nodularity of the uterus and tenderness of the adnexa. Pain is due to bleeding from ectopic endometrium. Almost 50% of patients with endometriosis are infertile.

PPx: None

MoD: Ectopic endometrial tissue forms on or beneath the pelvic mucosal/serosal surfaces → cyclic hyperplasia and degeneration due to response to female sex hormones → chronic hemorrhaging → **fibrotic pelvic adhesions** →infertility

Dx:
1. Pelvic exam (clinical diagnosis)
2. Beta-hCG
3. CBC, basic metabolic panel (BMP)
4. TVUS to r/o abnormal anatomy
5. Laparoscopy (will show chocolate-like material representing old blood) to confirm diagnosis

Tx/Mgmt:
1. NSAIDs ± combined OCPs
2. Progestins, GnRH agonists for those who don't respond to NSAIDs and OCPs
3. If no improvement → laparoscopy to biopsy, ablate, or excise implants

QUICK TIPS

The 3 Ds of endometriosis:
Dyschezia (pain when defecating) + Dysmenorrhea + Dyspareunia

Endometriosis, APGO video

4. Danazol if refractory to laparoscopy
5. Hysterectomy + bilateral salpingoophorectomy = definitive treatment

Pelvic Pain

There are many etiologies of pelvic pain, including some that are medical (e.g., diverticulitis causing left lower quadrant [LLQ] pain, appendicitis causing right lower quadrant [RLQ] pain, irritable bowel syndrome [IBS] causing chronic pelvic pain). Mittelschmerz and ovarian/adnexal torsion are two high-yield nonmalignant gynecologic causes for the shelf. Potential malignant causes of pelvic pain, such as cysts of the ovaries, are covered in Chapter 5. Ectopic pregnancy is covered in Chapter 14. PID is covered in Chapter 4.

Mittelschmerz

Buzz Words: Midcycle lower abdominal pain + normal ultra-sound+ normal history and physical (H&P)

Clinical Presentation: Patients with mittelschmerz experience pain halfway between their menstrual cycles due to normal follicular enlargement prior to ovulation. This is common in patients who ovulate normally and is NOT pathologic. As long as the pelvic ultrasound is normal, reassurance is all that is needed for treatment.

PPx: Avoid exposure to unopposed estrogen

MoD: Pain from normal follicular enlargement prior to ovulation

Dx:
1. Pelvic exam
2. Pelvic ultrasound

Tx/Mgmt:
1. Reassurance; no treatment needed

Ovarian/Adnexal Torsion

Buzz Words:
- **Acute intermittent abdominal pain** + last menstrual period (LMP) 6 weeks earlier with irregular menses + pelvic exam deferred for discomfort + **history of adnexal mass** + impaired ovarian blood flow → torsion of ovarian cyst
- Sudden onset pelvic pain (usually R-sided) + unilateral adnexal mass + nausea and vomiting (N/V) + low-grade fever → ovarian/adnexal torsion
- Sudden onset severe unilateral abdominal pain **following physical activity** + free fluid near ovarian cyst → ruptured ovarian cyst

Clinical Presentation: Ovarian or adnexal torsion is a surgical emergency. This disorder must be ruled out before more benign causes of pelvic pain (e.g., mittelschmerz) can be considered. Patients with masses in the ovary or fallopian tube are more likely to suffer from torsion.

In addition, be sure to rule out ovarian cyst rupture, which occurs in the setting of **physical activity.** Ovarian/adnexal torsion, on the other hand, can occur without physical activity.

PPx: Avoid risk factors such as pregnancy, ovulation during infertility treatment, ovarian masses >5 cm.

MoD: Partial or complete torsion of the ovary around the infundibulopelvic (suspensory) ligament of the ovary and the utero-ovarian ligaments. More commonly right-sided because left rectosigmoid colon occupies space around the left ovary.

- **Ovarian torsion** = partial or complete rotation of the ovary around the induibulopelvic (suspensory ligament of the ovary) and utero-ovarian ligaments
- **Adnexal torsion** = fallopian tube also twisting along with the ovary

Dx:
1. Pelvic exam
2. Beta-hCG to exclude ectopic pregnancy
3. Pelvic ultrasound (shows edematous ovary and **impaired ovarian blood flow**)
4. CBC and BMP

Tx/Mgmt:
1. Laparoscopic surgery for detorsion
2. Salpingo-oophorectomy for obvious adnexal necrosis or suspected ovarian malignancy

GUNNER PRACTICE

1. A 16-year-old female high school student presents to student health because of pelvic pain, nausea, and vomiting that keeps her from being able to concentrate in class. The symptoms began the day before, at the onset of menses, and have been alleviated only mildly by ibuprofen. She has experienced severe pelvic pain once every 30 days since she was 12, and each episode seems to correspond with an episode of menses. She has not sought medical advice about this previously because she was told by her parents that this pain was "normal" and that it "would pass." She denies abnormal vaginal bleeding or bleeding between menstrual cycles and does not take any regular medications. Although she recently acquired a boyfriend, she has never been sexually active. Her vital signs are within normal limits. On exam, she does not have tenderness with palpation of the lower abdomen, and her pelvic exam shows no abnormalities. What is the most likely diagnosis?

A. Normal menses

B. Primary dysmenorrhea

C. Premenstrual syndrome

D. Pelvic inflammatory disease from sexually transmitted infection

E. Adenomyosis

2. A 29-year-old, gravida 0, para 0, female comes to her Ob/Gyn care provider complaining of dull pelvic pain on the left side. The pain has been ongoing for the last 2 months and is exacerbated during menses. She has regular 28-day cycles; her last menstrual period began 2 weeks earlier. She reports being otherwise healthy and never needing to take any medication. Her 60-year-old mother was recently diagnosed with stage 1 breast cancer and has been receiving appropriate treatment. The patient works as a manager for a construction company and denies any recent traumatic injury. Her vital signs are 110/70 mmHg, 98.6 F, 80 bpm and 12 RR. On exam, there is tenderness to palpation of the left adnexa. Labs were ordered and a urine pregnancy test was found to be negative. A follow-up pelvic ultrasound shows a simple 4-cm cyst in her left ovary. Which of the following is the most appropriate next step in management?

A. Laparoscopy

B. Laparoscopy and removal of left ovary

C. Needle aspiration of the cyst

D. Danazol

E. Oral contraceptive pills and follow-up in 6 weeks

3. A previously healthy 20-year-old, gravida 0, para 0, female college student comes to the physician for pelvic pain that occurs once a month. Her menses occur in regular 28-day cycles and are associated with occasional pain and abdominal discomfort that does not disrupt her studies. However, around 2 weeks after her menses, she experiences a sharp pain on the left side of her lower abdomen. Although it is self-limiting, it gives her great discomfort as long as it lasts. She is otherwise healthy and does not take any medications. She denies alcohol and drug use. She has been sexually active with one partner and always uses condoms for protection. Her vitals are 110/70 mm Hg, 98.6° F, 80 bpm, and 20 RR. On exam, she does not have tenderness to palpation of her lower

abdomen, adnexa, or uterus. Her pelvic exam shows no abnormalities and a urine pregnancy test is normal. What is the next best step in managing this patient?

A. Transabdominal pelvic ultrasound
B. Transvaginal pelvic ultrasound
C. Culture and Gram stain to look for *Chlamydia trachomatis* and *Neisseria gonorrhoeae*
D. Reassurance
E. Pap smear

ANSWERS: What Would Gunner Jess/Jim Do?

1. WWGJD? A 16-year-old female high school student presents to student health because of pelvic pain, nausea and vomiting that keeps her from being able to concentrate in class. The symptoms began yesterday at the onset of menses and have only been mildly alleviated by ibuprofen. She has experienced cyclic, severe pelvic pain once every 30-day since she was 12, and each episode seems to correspond with an episode of menses. She has not sought medical advice about this previously because she was told by her parents that this pain was "normal" and that it "will pass." She denies vaginal bleeding or bleeding in between menstrual cycles and does not take any regular medications. Although she recently got a boyfriend, she has never been sexually active. Her vital signs are within normal limits. On exam, she does not have tenderness with palpation of the lower abdomen, and her pelvic exam shows no abnormalities. What is the most likely diagnosis?

Answer: B. Primary dysmenorrhea

Explanation: The patient's young age, painful menses that disrupt her routine, and normal pelvic exam all point to primary dysmenorrhea, which is a disorder characterized by debilitating pelvic pain during menses. Primary dysmenorrhea often peaks on the second day, which is what we see in this question stem. It is important to differentiate this from other closely related disorders on the differential for acute pelvic pain in young females, such as normal menses, premenstrual syndrome (PMS), and PID. On the shelf exam, normal menses would not disrupt a patient's normal activity, which is not the case here. PMS, on the other hand, would present with more generalized symptoms, such as mood disturbance or breast tenderness, which are not present in this patient. Finally, you can absolutely rule out PID because the question stem states that the patient has never been sexually active. Although a patient's history is not always reliable in real life, everything stated on the shelf can be treated as a fact.

A. Normal menses → Incorrect. Pelvic pain from normal menses on the shelf would not debilitate the patient.

C. Premenstrual syndrome → Incorrect. PMS on the shelf is associated with more systemic signs and symptoms, such as breast tenderness and abdominal bloating. Their onset is also often a day or so before menses.

D. Pelvic inflammatory disease from sexually transmitted infection → Incorrect. Patient has never been
sexually active. Remember to assume that everything written in the question stem is fact.
E. Adenomyosis → Incorrect. Patients with adenomyosis would present with a uniformly enlarged
soft, boggy uterus. Adenomyosis is the growth of
endometrial glands within the myometrium, leading
to pelvic pain during menses.

2. WWGJD? A 29-year-old, gravida 0, para 0, female
comes to her Ob/Gyn care provider complaining of
dull pelvic pain on the left side. The pain has been
ongoing for the last 2 months and is exacerbated during menses. She has regular 28-day cycles with her
last menstrual period being 2 weeks ago. She reports
being otherwise healthy and never needing to take any
medication. Her 60-year-old mother was recently diagnosed with stage 1 breast cancer and has been receiving appropriate treatment. She works as a manager for
a construction company and denies any recent traumatic injury. Her vital signs are 110/70 mm Hg, 98.6°
F, 80 bpm and 12 RR. On exam, there is tenderness
to palpation of the left adnexa. Labs were ordered and
a urine pregnancy test was found to be negative. A
follow-up pelvic ultrasound shows a simple, 4-cm cyst
in her left ovary. Which of the following is the most
appropriate next step in management?

Answer: E. Oral contraceptive pills and follow-up in 6 weeks
Explanation: This patient presents with a simple cyst
in her left ovary that is likely to be a functional
ovarian cyst. The biggest giveaway is that the ultrasound found it to be a simple instead of a complex
cyst; if it were complex, it would suggest an endometrioma. The second most likely diagnosis in this
question is endometriosis, which is characterized
by the appearance of endometrial tissue outside of
the uterus. Endometriosis classically presents with
the 3 Ds: dysmenorrhea, dyschezia, and dyspareunia. The patient in this scenario is less likely
to have dysmenorrhea because of an absence
of dyschezia/dyspareunia and the presence of a
simple cyst.

Unlike endometriosis, functional cysts are treated with
OCPs and a repeat pelvic exam in 6 weeks. The
OCPs are used to prevent ovulation and thus limit
the pelvic pain, which strikes whenever the ovary is
hormonally stimulated.

A. Laparoscopy → Incorrect. This would be the correct answer for further evaluation of the endometriosis, but it is more likely that patient has a functional cyst.

B. Laparoscopy and removal of the left ovary → Incorrect. Again, removal of the left ovary at this point is premature. B can be ruled out since it is the most invasive.

C. Needle aspiration of the cyst → Incorrect. A simple cyst can be observed and does not need to be further evaluated at this point.

D. Danazol → Incorrect. Danazol is the treatment for endometriosis only if the patient is refractory to laparoscopy.

3. WWGJD? A previously healthy 20-year-old, gravida 0, para 0, female college student comes to the physician for pelvic pain that occurs once a month. Her menses occurs at regular 28-day cycles and is associated with occasional pain and abdominal discomfort that does not disrupt her studies. However, around 2 weeks after her menses, she experiences a sharp pain on the left side of her lower abdomen. Although it is self-limiting, it gives her great discomfort throughout the pain's duration. She is otherwise healthy and does not take any medications. She denies alcohol and drug use. She has been sexually active with one partner and always uses condoms for protection. Her vitals are 110/70 mm Hg, 98.6° F, 80 bpm, and 20 RR. On exam, she does not have tenderness to palpation of her lower abdomen, adnexa, or uterus. Her pelvic exam shows no abnormalities and a urine pregnancy test is normal. What is the next best step in managing this patient?

Answer: D. Reassurance

Explanation: The patient in this question stem has Mittelschmerz, which is characterized by pain during ovulation (e.g., 14 days or 2 weeks after a menstrual period). Aside from the brief discomfort, it is benign and does not lead to further pathology. It also typically does not force patients to miss work. Treatment is just reassurance that the symptoms are benign. Other frequently seen causes of pelvic pain in a young female are sexually transmitted infections (STIs), functional ovarian cysts, endometrioma, and pregnancy.

A. Transabdominal pelvic ultrasound → Incorrect. This could be used to look for endometriosis or a functional ovarian cyst. It would be a better treatment option if the patient's pain occurred during menses.

B. Transvaginal pelvic ultrasound → Incorrect. This could be used to look for endometriosis or a functional ovarian cyst. It would be a better treatment option if the patient's pain occurred during menses.

C. Culture and Gram stain to look for *Chlamydia trachomatis* and *Neisseria gonorrhoeae* → Incorrect. Although she is sexually active, the patient's risk of transmission is less likely with protection. In addition, *Chlamydia* and gonorrhea do not require a diagnostic test before they can be treated.

E. Pap smear → Incorrect. The age to begin Pap smear screenings is 21 years.

Sexual Dysfunction

Kumar Nadhan, Hao-Hua Wu, and Leo Wang

GUNNER COLUMN

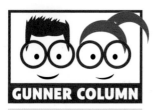

99 AR

When sex is painful ACOG FAQ

99 AR

AAFP dyspareunia differential

MNEMONIC

Dyspareunia differential = DATIVE
Domestic Abuse, Atropic Vaginitis,
Tumor, Infection, Vaginismus,
Endometriosis

QUICK TIPS

"Positional" pain often refers to
inflammation of an organ deep in
the pelvis, as with endometriosis
or cystitis.

Introduction

Sexual dysfunction is a sensitive topic for patients. It includes any difficulty with sexual experiences. All conditions within this broad category carry physical and psychological implications, both of which must be addressed in treatment.

The disorders covered in the chapter appear only occasionally on the shelf and are more useful to know for your clinical rotation. An important organizing principle is to be sure to rule out sexually transmitted infections (STIs) in evaluating these patients.

Buzz Words: Painful intercourse + fear of intercourse + sexual abuse + history of STIs + perimenopausal woman

Clinical Presentation: Broadly, dyspareunia is pain associated with sexual intercourse. This may be physiologic or psychologically induced pain that localizes in the external genitalia (in a patient <50 years old) or deep within the pelvis (in a patient >50 years old). Postmenopausal women may experience the pain because of vaginal atrophy, discussed in Chapter 7. The pain may not be limited to the time of sexual intercourse but may present before or after the event.

Dyspareunia is often chronic and can be associated with interstitial cystitis, *Candida* infection (excoriations caused by itching), hypoestrogenic states such as menopause, urethral diverticula, and endometriosis.

Prophylaxis (PPx): N/A

Mechanism of Disease (MoD):

- Congenital anatomic malformation → pain with first tampon
- Inflammation/infection
- Perimenopause → decreased estrogen → vaginal atrophy

Diagnostic Steps (Dx):

1. Sexual history (rule out abuse) and pelvic exam
2. Beta-human chorionic gonadotropin (beta-hCG) if of reproductive age
3. Urinalysis (UA)/urine culture (UCx)
4. Tests to r/o STIs (e.g., wet mount for *Candida*, etc.)

Treatment and Management Steps (Tx/Mgmt):

1. Variable, based on underlying cause

- Adequate lubrication
- Lidocaine ointment
- Clear infection/inflammation

Orgasmic Dysfunction

Buzz Words: Delayed/no orgasm + anxiety + depression + problems in relationship

Clinical Presentation: Orgasmic dysfunction is approached mainly as a psychological phenomenon in which a female has delayed or absent orgasm despite sufficient sexual stimulation. Such patients may have a history of anxiety or depression.

PPx: N/A

MoD: Multifactorial, psychosocial elements

Dx:
1. Sexual history (rule out abuse) and pelvic exam
2. Beta-hCG if of reproductive age
3. UA/UCx
4. Tests to r/o STIs (e.g., wet mount for *Candida*, etc.)

Tx/Mgmt:
1. Assessment of how patient views and experiences sex, relationships.
2. Refer to psychiatrist if no functional pathology found.

Persistent Sexual Arousal Syndrome

Buzz Words: Postmenopausal female + inability to function normally + constant arousal + multiple orgasms daily

Clinical Presentation: Persistent sexual arousal syndrome (PSAS) is a very rare syndrome that manifests as persistent and uncontrollable genital arousal independent of sexual desire. PSAS is a poorly understood condition that can severely affect concentration and relationships in everyday life.

PSAS case report

PPx: N/A

MoD: Unknown

Dx:
1. Sexual history and pelvic exam

Tx/Mgmt:
1. Psychotherapy
2. SSRIs

Vaginismus

Buzz Words:
- Pain with tampons/sexual intercourse + fear of penetration

- First sexual experience + "sex is taboo" upbringing + tense perineal musculature + pain upon penetration + everything else normal

Clinical Presentation: Vaginismus includes any pain, psychological or physical, associated with vaginal penetration (does not have to be sexual; can result from tampon insertion). Patients with highly sheltered or religious upbringing may be more likely to have vaginismus.

PPx: N/A

MoD: Unknown, but the end result is an involuntary spasm of the outer third of the vagina, which interferes with sex. Spasms can also occur with tampon insertion.

Dx:

1. Sexual history (r/o abuse) and pelvic exam

Tx/Mgmt:

1. Desensitization using dilators to help patient control pelvic floor muscles
2. Kegel and relaxation exercises
3. Sex therapy

GUNNER PRACTICE

1. A 56-year-old woman comes to your office for an annual checkup. She has a history of breast cancer treated with a partial mastectomy as well as hypertension and a 30 pack-year history of smoking. She has also recently lost 30 pounds, feels more confident, and has seen a resurgence of her libido. She has been dating a man for the last month and has begun having sexual intercourse, but experiences burning pain after a minute of penetration. What is the best first step in management?
   A. Evaluate history of STI
   B. Pregnancy test
   C. Ask about use of vaginal lubrication
   D. Computed tomography (CT) abdomen/pelvis
   E. Advise to quit smoking

Notes

ANSWER: What Would Gunner Jess/Jim Do?

1. WWGJD? A 56-year-old woman comes to your office for an annual checkup. She has a history of breast cancer treated with a partial mastectomy, hypertension, and 30 pack-year history of smoking. She has also recently lost 30 pounds, feels more confident, and has seen a resurgence of her libido. She has been dating a man for the last month and **has begun having sexual intercourse, but experiences burning pain after a minute of penetration. What is the best first step in management?**

Answer: C. Ask about use of vaginal lubrication

Explanation: The most common cause of dyspareunia in postmenopausal women is vaginal atrophy. The pain is most likely due to intense friction, alleviated by lubrication.

A. Evaluate history of sexually transmitted infections (STIs) → Incorrect. Burning pain is often associated with a sexually transmitted infection; however, this pain occurs only during sexual penetration. This is most likely dyspareunia.

B. Pregnancy test→ Incorrect. Although pregnancy should be of concern in most cases of sexual dysfunction, the patient's age and symptoms point to dyspareunia.

D. CT abdomen/pelvis → Incorrect. Imaging is not recommended in early evaluation of dyspareunia.

E. Advise to quit smoking → Incorrect. Quitting smoking is always a good suggestion to patients. In this case it does not help the patient's primary concern, which should be addressed first.

Traumatic and Mechanical Disorders

Hao-Hua Wu and Leo Wang

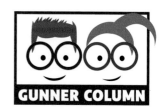

Introduction

Traumatic and mechanical disorders comprise conditions that occur either through external injury or through weakening of the physical support system for the urinary, reproductive, and terminal gastrointestinal (GI) tracts. Disorders such as Asherman syndrome and pelvic organ prolapse (of the uterus/vagina) are favorites of the National Board of Medical Examiners (NBME). Ovarian torsion and urinary incontinence are also high-yield because they are in the differential for common chief complaints (e.g., abdominal pain and urinary frequency/urgency, respectively), which allows them to be tested on other exams, such as the Medicine and Surgery shelf exams. The most important organizing principle in this chapter is to understand the mechanism of disease, which is usually straightforward and will tell you exactly what signs/symptoms to expect.

This chapter is organized into (1) Traumatic Disorders, (2) Mechanical Disorders, and (3) Gunner Practice. Anticipate spending 4 to 6 hours for the first and second pass.

Traumatic Disorders

The only traumatic disorder that is high-yield is Asherman syndrome. Other direct insults that lead directly to traumatic injury to the reproductive system are injuries, burns, and sexual intercourse. These are rarely tested; if they are, the etiology is usually obvious (e.g., car crash, recent burn, recent sexual intercourse leading to vaginal bleeding/pain).

Asherman Syndrome

Buzz Words: Amenorrhea + history of **dilatation and curettage (D&C)** to treat postpartum hemorrhage + negative beta-human chorionic gonadotropin (beta-hCG) + progestin challenge has no withdrawal bleeding + follicle-stimulating hormone/thyroid-stimulating hormone (FSH/TSH)/prolactin within normal limits

Clinical Presentation: Asherman syndrome is a disorder defined by the presence of intrauterine adhesions (IUAs) that cause infertility and amenorrhea. Patients classically present with either amenorrhea or inability to become pregnant after a D&C procedure. The classic procedure on the shelf is a D&C to remove placenta accreta/increta/percreta and treat postpartum hemorrhage, although any surgical procedure of the endometrial lining (e.g., D&C to clear products of conception after spontaneous abortion) may cause it. This is a high-yield topic on the Ob/Gyn shelf, particularly with regard to secondary causes of amenorrhea. Be sure to rule out other causes of amenorrhea, such as pregnancy, endocrine defect, or Sheehan syndrome in the workup of these patients.

Prophylaxis (PPx):
- Avoid unnecessary surgical procedures to the uterine lining.
- Counsel patient in the event D&C is used for postpartum hemorrhage, removal of retained placenta, or treatment of incomplete/missed spontaneous abortion.

Mechanism of Disease (MoD): Traumatic injury to uterine lining due to instrumentation → scar tissue formation → IUAs → blockage

Diagnostic Steps (Dx):
1. Beta-hCG (negative)
2. FSH, TSH, prolactin (normal)
3. Progestin challenge to look for withdrawal bleed to r/o Sheehan
4. Hysteroscopy is the gold standard for diagnosis.
5. Hysterosalpingogram or hysterosonography can also be used to look for IUAs.

Treatment and Management Steps (Tx/Mgmt):
1. Hysteroscopy (lysis of adhesions) with estrogen postop to regenerate uterine lining

Mechanical Disorders

The muscles of the pelvic floor and associated muscles/fascia hold the bladder, vagina/cervix/uterus, and rectum in place. Weakening or disruption of these muscles leads to mechanical disorders such as pelvic organ prolapse, stress incontinence, or cystourethroceles. The most common signs and symptoms of mechanical disorders of the female reproductive tract involve the urinary, reproductive, and terminal GI tracts, such as urinary incontinence, pelvic pain/pressure/mass/dyspareunia, and constipation, respectively. The organizing principle here is that patients will complain of symptoms based on the organ affected. Keep a keen eye out for buzz words and how to differentiate these disorders, as they will be frequently tested.

Although not essential, a quick review of anatomy may help better understand these symptoms. The most high-yield anatomy to know (but not directly tested) is the following for the innervation of the bladder:

- Skeletal muscles of pelvic floor → pudendal nerve (S2-4)
- Beta-adrenergic receptors that cause the bladder to relax (e.g., inhibition of urination) → sympathetic nerves from T11–L2
- Alpha-adrenergic receptors at bladder neck (e.g., enable urination) → parasympathetic nerves to the intrinsic sphincter

General Mechanical Disorders

Pelvic Organ Prolapse

Buzz Words: Pelvic pressure and heaviness + mass protruding into vaginal wall outside vaginal cavity + gradual urinary incontinence + history of pelvic surgery

Clinical Presentation: Uterine prolapse, part of the constellation of pelvic organ prolapse, is the displacement of the uterus from its normal anatomic position inferiorly through the vaginal canal. The most common complaints are fullness, dyspareunia, and pelvic pressure at first with incontinence and constipation developing gradually over time. Uterine prolapse is graded by level of descent, but this classification is not tested on the shelf. Differentiate from vaginal prolapse through physical exam (e.g., vaginal-only vs. uterine prolapse, which contains both cervix and vagina).

PPx: Avoid risk factors like hysterectomies or prior pelvic procedures

MoD: Hysterectomy → weakening of pelvic floor musculature → uterine prolapse → compression on bladder/urethra → urinary incontinence

Dx:
1. Pelvic exam to look for mass in canal
2. Urinalysis (UA)/urine culture (UCx) (workup of urinary incontinence if concomitant)
3. Biopsy of vaginal/cervical ulcers to r/o cancer

Tx/Mgmt:
1. For uterine prolapse:
   - Supportive (for pain from ulcerations of prolapsed organ)
   - Pessaries
   - Kegel exercises
   - Colporrhaphy
   - Laparotomy/laparoscopy for hysterectomy
   - Treatment of urinary incontinence

99 AR

Video of total uterine prolapse

99 AR

Uterine prolapse grading scale

99 AR

Video of pessaries

99 AR

Colpocleisis = procedure that closes the vagina; used to treat vaginal prolapse. (Video)

QUICK TIPS

Prodentia (Latin for "to fall down") means falling down of an organ from usual anatomic position → increases risk for uterine or ureteral obstruction

99 AR

For cystocele repair → fix defects in pubocervical fascia and reattach to side wall/white arcus tendineus fascia (white line); Repair ONLY WHEN SYMPTOMATIC!

2. For vaginal prolapse:
   - Supportive (for pain from ulcerations of prolapsed organ)
   - Pessaries
   - Kegel exercises
   - Colporrhaphy
   - Repair of supporting vaginal cuff attached to sacrospinous and uterosacral ligaments
   - Colpocleisis if prodentia (vagina blocks urethra at apex)
   - Laparotomy/laparoscopy for hysterectomy
   - Treatment of urinary incontinence

Cystocele/Urethrocele

Buzz Words: Incontinence (stress, overflow, urge) + concomitant cystocele

Clinical Presentation: A urethrocele is the bulging of the urethra into the vaginal canal. It is often accompanied by cystocele in a disorder known as cystourethrocele. You won't be asked to differentiate cysto- and urethrocele from one another because they are difficult to distinguish, but you need to know how to compare them with recto- and enteroceles.

PPx: Avoid procedures of anterior vaginal canal

MoD: Weakening of anterior vaginal musculature/fascia

Dx:

1. Pelvic exam
2. UA/UCx (workup of incontinence)

Tx/Mgmt:

1. Supportive + treatment of urinary incontinence
2. Pessaries
3. Kegel exercises
4. Surgical management with colporrhaphy

Enterocele

Buzz Words: History of hysterectomy + pelvic pressure/fullness + mass protruding into posterior vaginal canal + mass enlarges with Valsalva

Clinical Presentation: An enterocele is a weakening of the vaginal canal that allows the protrusion of GI contents, such as the small intestine and peritoneum. It is associated with a past history of surgery that disrupted the levator ani. It is NOT associated with incontinence, unlike urethro- and cystoceles. It is a type of vaginal prolapse.

PPx: Avoid hysterectomies

MoD: Weakening of rectovaginal fascia and pubocervical fascia → GI contents protruding into vaginal canal

Dx:
1. P/E (diagnosis made clinically when protrusion felt on Valsalva)

Tx/Mgmt:
1. Supportive
2. Pessaries
3. Kegel exercises
4. Surgical management with colporrhaphy

Rectocele

Buzz Words: Constipation alleviated by pressure to posterior vaginal wall + past surgery that disrupted the levator ani + posterior vaginal canal mass enlarged by Valsalva → rectocele

Clinical Presentation: A rectocele is a weakening of the vaginal canal that allows the rectum to protrude. It is a type of vaginal prolapse.

PPx: Avoid constipation

MoD: Weakening of rectovaginal fascia and pubocervical fascia → rectum protrusion into vaginal canal

Dx:
1. P/E (diagnosis made clinically when protrusion felt on Valsalva); see Table 10.1

Tx/Mgmt:
1. Supportive treatment
2. Pessaries
3. Kegel exercises
4. Surgical management with colporrhaphy (repair rectovaginal fascia)

Imperforate Hymen

Buzz Words: Teenage female + cyclic lower abdominal pain + no menstruation + bluish mass protruding from vagina

99 AR
Colporrhaphy is a procedure that strengthens the vaginal canal with sutures.

TABLE 10.1 How to Differentiate Cystocele Versus Urethrocele Versus Enterocele Versus Rectocele

	Cystocele	Urethrocele	Enterocele	Rectocele
Definition	Protrusion of **bladder** into vaginal canal	Protrusion of **urethra** into vaginal canal	Protrusion of **GI contents** (small intestine/peritoneum) into vaginal canal	Protrusion of **rectum** into vaginal canal
Buzz words	Incontinence (stress, overflow, urge) + concomitant urethrocele	Incontinence (stress, overflow, urge) + concomitant cystocele	History of hysterectomy	Constipation alleviated by pressure to posterior vaginal wall

Clinical Presentation: Imperforate hymen is a common form of vaginal outflow obstruction that should be on the differential for amenorrhea. It presents in a teenage female who has yet to have her first period yet has cyclical abdominal pain (e.g. menstrual cycles). This means that the endometrium is shedding but the obstruction by the imperforate hymen prevents blood from getting out. Thus, on examination, a "bluish mass" is seen protruding from the vaginal canal.

PPx: N/A

MoD: Failure of hymen to involute

Dx:

1. Pelvic exam

Tx/Mgmt:

1. Surgical opening of vaginal canal to allow for menstruation

Ovarian Torsion

Buzz Words: Acute onset of unilateral lower abdominal pain + nausea/vomiting + unilateral tender adnexal mass on exam + pelvic ultrasound with Doppler showing enlarged ovary with decreased blood flow

Clinical Presentation: Ovarian torsion is a partial or complete rotation of the ovary around the infundibulopelvic and utero-ovarian ligaments. It should always be on the differential when lower abdominal pain in a female is being evaluated. If the fallopian tube is involved, then this is known as **adnexal torsion.** The larger the ovary grows, the greater the patient's risk of experiencing torsion. Thus torsion can sometimes be associated with cysts or benign tumors of the ovary.

PPx: Avoid risk factors such as pregnancy and ovarian enlargement due to cysts/benign tumors.

MoD: Partial or complete rotation of the ovary (or fallopian tube if adnexal) around the infundibulopelvic and utero-ovarian ligaments

Dx:

1. Pelvic exam
2. Transvaginal ultrasound (gold standard)

Tx/Mgmt:

1. Immediate surgical management to untwist ovary (and/or fallopian tube) and prevent necrosis

Urinary Incontinence

Urinary incontinence is the loss of bladder control and manifests as involuntary leakage. For the wards, you may hear urinary incontinence categorized as stress urinary incontinence vs. urgency urinary incontinence vs. mixed (see ACOG Practice Bulletin 155). However, the US

TABLE 10.2 Differentiating Among Etiologies for Urinary Incontinence

	Stress Incontinence	Continuous Incontinence	Urge Incontinence	Overflow Incontinence	Mixed Incontinence
Etiology	Mechanical	Mechanical	Neurogenic (hyperactive cholinergic)	Neurogenic (hypoactive cholinergic)	Mechanical— neurogenic
Buzz words	Increased urine loss with Valsalva	Urine dribbling from vagina	Nocturia, diabetes/multiple sclerosis	Urethral/bladder obstruction, high postvoid residual volume	Combination of stress and urge/overflow buzz words

Medical Licensing Examination (USMLE) Content Outline and the NBME questions contain an older categorization of urinary incontinence that also includes continuous and overflow incontinence. Thus this chapter covers the latter.

Although only two types of urinary incontinence (stress and continuous) can be considered mechanical disorders, the other types (overflow and urge) are important to know in order to narrow down the differential on the shelf.

The most important organizing principle is that every type of urinary incontinence should be evaluated when the chief complaint is urinary frequency, urgency, hesitancy, or "leaking urine." See Table 10.2 for an overview.

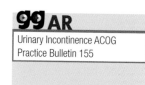

99 AR

Urinary Incontinence ACOG Practice Bulletin 155

Stress Incontinence

Buzz Words: Drainpipe urethra (means internal sphincter is not working) + immobile urethra + constant leakage of urine + no fistula found + leakage of urine w/Valsalva (e.g., laughing) → intrinsic sphincter deficiency

Clinical Presentation: Stress incontinence occurs when the urethral sphincter is "stressed," most commonly by Valsalva maneuvers (e.g., coughing, sneezing, laughing, running).

PPx: Avoid risk factors: pregnancy, unnecessary pelvic surgery, obesity, diuresis-causing meds/drugs (e.g., caffeine)

MoD:
- Weakness of pelvic floor muscles → weak sphincter → urethral hypermobility → neck of bladder is displaced → pressure on bladder > pressure on urethra → urine leakage
- Advanced age/inadequate estrogen levels/previous surgery → intrinsic urethral sphincter deficiency → urine leakage

Dx:
1. History and physical (H&P): r/o medication cause (e.g., diuretics, caffeine); pelvic exam to look for signs of pelvic floor muscle weakness, such as uterine prolapse or cystocele

99 AR

Types of urinary incontinence video

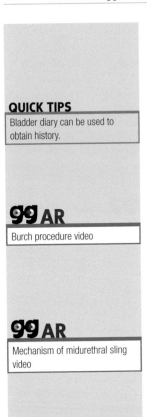

2. UA/UCx (normal)
3. Cystometry (normal); evaluate with cystoureteroscopy if hematuria is present
4. Postvoid residual volume (normal)
5. Cough stress test (seeing urine leak out of urethra during cough)
6. Urethral cotton swab (diagnostic if >30 degree angle with increased intra-abdominal pressure)

Tx/Mgmt:
1. Kegel exercises
2. Pessaries
3. Estrogen replacement (in postmenopausal patient)
4. Pseudoephedrine (alpha-adrenergic properties maintain urethral tone versus surgery) → Burch procedure (a type of **retropubic urethropexy**) versus synthetic midurethral sling procedure versus **urethral bulking** (for internal sphincter deficiency)

Continuous Incontinence

Buzz Words: Urine from vagina instead of urethra + history of recent procedure

Clinical Presentation: Continuous incontinence is urinary incontinence caused by a genitourinary fistula (continuous leakage of urine); presents in a patient who had recent procedure or pregnancy and is dribbling urine from the vagina. Shelf will only test you on identifying the disease (buzz words).

Urge Incontinence (aka Overactive Bladder)

Buzz Words: Urinary incontinence due to uncontrollable desire to void + large loss of urine + nocturia (getting up in the middle of night to pee) + urinary frequency → urge incontinence

Clinical Presentation: Urge incontinence is **not** a mechanical disorder and is rather caused by irritation of the nerves that lead to irregular and uninhibited bladder contractions. Common chief complaint is urinary frequency and urgency. Differentiate this from stress incontinence by the nocturia buzz word. Also, leakage of urine is not associated with increased intra-abdominal pressure.

PPx: Oxybutynin

MoD:
- Detrusor instability due to overactive anticholinergic receptors
- Bladder irritation from neoplasm
- Interstitial cystitis

Dx:
1. Pelvic exam to look for signs of pelvic floor muscle weakness such as uterine prolapse or cystocele
2. UA/UCx (normal)
3. Cystometrogram (uninhibited contraction of bladder with filling)

Tx/Mgmt:
1. Oxybutynin (anticholinergic to decrease detrusor instability)

Overflow Incontinence

Buzz Words: Long history of **uncontrolled diabetes** + dribbling urine + high postvoid residual volume

Clinical Presentation: Overflow incontinence is also a nonmechanical cause of urinary incontinence. However, unlike urge incontinence, it is the result of parasympathetic denervation and impaired contractility of the bladder. The key buzz word is the association of diabetes or multiple sclerosis (e.g., neuropathies) with overflow incontinence. Thus the only way urine can leak is when the bladder fills up with so much fluid that the bladder pressure overcomes the strength of the internal and external sphincters and urine leaks through until the pressure is equalized. This type of incontinence is also associated with **obstruction** from prolapse or cysto-/urethroceles.

PPx: Treat obstruction

MoD:
- Postoperative state (including nerve injury due to childbirth)
- Epidural anesthesia
- **Diabetic** neuropathy
- Multiple sclerosis
- Stroke

Dx:
1. Pelvic exam to look for signs of pelvic floor muscle weakness to r/o stress in continence
2. UA/UCx (normal)
3. Postvoid residual (high)

Tx/Mgmt:
1. Intermittent catheterization
2. Bethanechol (activates muscarinic receptors)
3. Alpha blockers

Mixed Incontinence

Buzz Words: Leakage of urine due to increased intra-abdominal pressure + nocturia + hypercontractility of bladder

Clinical Presentation: Mixed incontinence is urinary incontinence that involves aspects of both urge and stress incontinence (e.g., detrusor instability and pelvic wall weakness combined). The shelf will test you only on identifying the disease (buzz words).

GUNNER PRACTICE

1. A 33-year-old, gravida 1, para 0, woman at 28 weeks' gestation presents to the OB triage unit with vaginal bleeding. The bright red blood has increased in volume since the patient noticed it an hour earlier. She reports no other symptoms and denies pelvic or abdominal pain. She and her significant other last had unprotected sexual intercourse 12 hours earlier, and neither has any history of sexually transmitted infections. Since becoming pregnant, she has had intermittent nausea that waxes and wanes. Otherwise the pregnancy has been uncomplicated and her last ultrasound 8 weeks earlier showed the placenta to be intact. Her vitals are 110/70 mm Hg, 99°F, 14 RR, 80 bpm, and 95% on room air. Exam shows no abdominal or uterine tenderness and a closed cervical os. Fundal height is 28 cm and fetal heart rate is 160/min. On monitoring of the fetus, there are two contractions per hour. What is the most likely diagnosis?
   A. Spontaneous abortion
   B. Placenta previa
   C. Sexually transmitted infection (STI)
   D. Cervical neoplasm
   E. Cervical trauma

2. A 60-year-old, gravida 2, para 2, woman comes to the physician because of a 5-month history of "leaking urine." She complains that it has been hard to control her urge to urinate; she has wet her pants in public so many times that she now wears a pad whenever she leaves the house. The loss of urine is not associated with laughing or bearing down. Five times a week, she will wake up in the middle of the night to urinate. Urination is not associated with pain, hesitancy, or blood. She has a history of fibroids but is otherwise healthy. Her vital signs are 98.6°F, 120/80 mm Hg, 70 bpm, and 14 RR. Exam reveals no costovertebral or uterine tenderness. Urinalysis and urine culture show no abnormalities. Ultrasound of the pelvis shows a 2-cm anterior mass within the musculature of the uterus. What is the most likely mechanism of her symptoms?

A. Leiomyoma uteri
B. Urinary tract infection
C. Detrusor instability
D. Higher pressure in the bladder compared with the urethra
E. Retention of urine in the bladder with overflow into the urethra

3. A 61-year-old woman, gravida 1, para 1, comes to the physician complaining of a mass in the vaginal canal. Patient states that she has been experiencing pressure in the lower abdomen and pelvic region for 3 months and that these symptoms are exacerbated after prolonged standing when she is at work as a teacher. She denies any dysuria, urinary urgency/frequency, or changes in bowel movement. Her past surgical history is significant for a hysterectomy. Her vital signs are 99°F, 130/90 mm Hg, 80 bpm, and 12 RR. On exam, there is a soft mass on the superoposterior wall of the vagina that enlarges when the patient coughs. Otherwise there is no tenderness to pelvic or abdominal palpation. Surgical scar is clean, dry, and intact. Urinalysis shows no evidence of infection. What is the most likely diagnosis?
A. Enterocele
B. Uretocele
C. Cystocele
D. Rectocele
E. Vaginal tumor

ANSWERS: What Would Gunner Jess/Jim Do?

1. WWGJD? A 33-year-old, gravid 1, para 0, woman is at 28 weeks' gestation and presents to the OB triage unit with vaginal bleeding. The bright red blood has increased in volume since the patient noticed it an hour ago. She reports no other symptoms and denies pelvic or abdominal pain. She and her significant other last had unprotected sexual intercourse 12 hours ago, and neither has any history of sexually transmitted infections. Since becoming pregnant, she has had intermittent nausea that waxes and wanes. Otherwise, the pregnancy has been uncomplicated and her last ultrasound 8 weeks ago showed the placenta intact. Her vitals are 110/70 mm Hg, 99°F, 14 RR, 80 bpm and 95% on room air. Exam shows no abdominal or uterine tenderness and closed cervical external os. Fundal height is 28 cm and fetal heart rate is 160/min. Two contractions per hour are shown with monitoring of the fetus. What is the most likely diagnosis?

Answer: E. Cervical trauma

> Explanation: In this question, a woman at 28 weeks' gestation presents with vaginal bleeding 12 hours after sex. An important organizing principle is that the most recent thing that happened to a patient (e.g., newly described drug, most recent pertinent event such as sexual intercourse for vaginal bleeding) is most likely the etiology of an **acute chief complaint.** In this question stem, the clue of sexual intercourse that immediately preceded the symptoms makes it likely that this patient is suffering from cervical trauma. She and her fetus are otherwise healthy and do not exhibit any other signs of pathology.
>
> A. Spontaneous abortion → Incorrect. By definition, spontaneous abortion is loss of fetus within the first 20 weeks of gestation. The fact that this woman is at 28 weeks' gestation rules this answer choice out immediately.
>
> B. Placenta previa → Incorrect. Placenta previa refers to the condition where the placenta is blocking part or all of the uterine neck, thus interfering with delivery. This would usually be spotted on ultrasound and was noted here.
>
> C. STI → Incorrect. This answer may be tempting given that "unprotected" was thrown in the question stem to confuse readers. However, the fact that patient and significant other are stated to not have STIs makes this less likely.

D. Cervical neoplasm → Incorrect. Sometimes a patient with a cervical neoplasm can develop bleeding, often from the site of the neoplasm. It is unclear here because this diagnosis is confirmed with an imaging.

2. **WWGJD?** A 60-year-old, gravida 2, para 2, woman comes to the physician because of a **5-month history of "leaking urine."** She complains that it has been hard to control her urge to urinate and has wet her pants in public so many times that she now wears a pad whenever leaving the house. The loss of urine is not associated with laughing or bearing down. Five times a week, she will wake up in the middle of the night to urinate. Urination is not associated with pain, hesitancy, or blood. She has a history of fibroids, but is otherwise healthy. Her vital signs are 98.6°F, 120/80 mm Hg, 70 bpm, and 14 RR. Exam reveals no costovertebral nor uterine tenderness. Urinalysis and urine culture show no abnormalities. Ultrasound of pelvis shows a 2-cm anterior mass within the musculature of the uterus. What can the physician say is the most likely mechanism of her symptoms?

Answer: C. Detrusor instability

Explanation: This patient likely has urinary incontinence (aka "leaking urine") due to detrusor instability because of two important clues: (1) loss of urine is not associated with increased intra-abdominal pressure (laughing or Valsalva) and (2) the feeling of urgency wakes her up at night. The first clue rules out stress incontinence and the second clue points to a hyperactive bladder rather than a hypoactive one, which would lead to retention of urine. Don't be fooled by the "anterior mass" in the uterus, which is a fibroid, as suggested by the patient's past medical history. Fibroids contained within the musculature of the uterus are typically not big enough to lead to incontinence by mass effect on the bladder. Treatment of detrusor instability is with medication.

A. Leiomyoma uteri → Incorrect. Leiomyoma uteri, aka fibroids, in this case are inside the myometrium of the uterus and well encapsulated and small enough (2 cm) to have no mass effect on the bladder, even though located anteriorly.

B. Urinary tract infection → Incorrect. Negative UA and UCx effectively rule out urinary tract infection (UTI) on the shelf.

D. Higher pressure in the bladder compared with the urethra → Incorrect. This is the mechanism of stress incontinence and is associated with urine leakage in the setting of increased intra-abdominal pressure, which is not seen in this scenario.

E. Retention of urine in the bladder with overflow into the urethra → Incorrect. This is the mechanism for retention incontinence, in which the bladder cannot contract, leading to leakage of the urine through the internal and external sphincter when fluid level reaches a critical volume. The clue that makes this less likely is the fact that patient's urgency wakes her up at night.

3. **WWGJD?** A 61-year-old woman, gravida 1, para 1, comes to the physician complaining of a mass in the vaginal canal. Patient states that she has been experiencing pressure in the lower abdomen and pelvic region for the past 3 months and that these symptoms are exacerbated after prolonged standing when at work as a teacher. She denies any dysuria, urinary urgency/frequency or changes in bowel movement. Her past surgical history is significant for a hysterectomy. Her vital signs are 99°F, 130/90 mm Hg, 80 bpm, and 12 RR. On exam, there is a soft mass that is present on the superior posterior wall of the vagina that enlarges when the patient coughs. Otherwise there is no tenderness to pelvic or abdominal palpation. Surgical scar is clean, dry, and intact. Urinalysis shows no evidence of infection. What is the most likely diagnosis?

Answer: A. Enterocele

Explanation: The clues in this question stem point to enterocele, which is a bulging of either the small intestine or peritoneum into the vaginal canal. The three buzz words that suggest enterocele are (1) history of hysterectomy, (2) posterior mass of vaginal canal (as opposed to anterior mass for cystocele), and (3) no constipation or urinary urgency/frequency (r/o recto-, cysto- and uretoceles, respectively). Enteroceles are evaluated and diagnosed clinically and treated by pessaries, Kegel exercises, and surgical management (e.g., colporrhaphy).

B. Urethrocele → Incorrect. Uretocele is the bulging of the urethra into the vaginal canal. This would present as an anterior mass with urinary incontinence and is associated with concomitant cystocele. The lack of urinary incontinence symptoms makes this diagnosis less likely.

C. Cystocele → Incorrect. Cystocele is the bulging of the bladder into the vaginal canal. This would

present as an anterior mass with urinary incontinence and is associated with concomitant urethrocele. The lack of urinary incontinence symptoms
makes this diagnosis less likely.
D. Rectocele → Incorrect. Rectocele is the bulging of
the rectum into the vaginal canal. This would present as posterior mass with constipation. The lack of
constipation (or changes in bowel movement) make
this diagnosis less likely.
E. Vaginal tumor → Incorrect. Unlikely to be a neoplasm because the mass can grow or shrink based
on Valsalva maneuver. A vaginal tumor would
be the same size regardless of intra-abdominal
pressure.

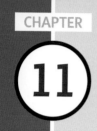

Congenital Disorders

Kumar Nadhan, Hao-Hua Wu, and Leo Wang

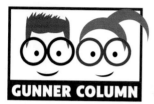

11

GUNNER COLUMN

Introduction

The complexity of the female reproductive tract increases the likelihood of congenital disorders, as there are several points in development that may develop aberrantly. Luckily for us, these disorders are easily distinguishable and recognizable. Note that the paramensoenphric duct is also known as the müllerian duct; that is, the two terms are synonymous and are used interchangeably. This chapter is high-yield for your Pediatrics shelf as well. Additionally, cervical insufficiency is a topic that frequently appears on the Ob/Gyn shelf, as it is on the differential for any pregnant woman who experiences preterm labor.

Müllerian Agenesis

QUICK TIPS

Absent secondary sex characteristics points to androgen insensitivity syndrome (AIS)

Buzz Words: Primary amenorrhea + normal secondary sex characteristics + normal 46XX karyotype

Clinical Presentation: A young female (between 8 and 18 years of age) has normal breast growth and pubic hair but has not yet experienced menarche. Her mother was exposed to diethylstilbestrol (DES) during pregnancy.

Prophylaxis (PPx): N/A

Mechanism of Disease (MoD): The müllerian (paramesonephric) ducts normally develop into the fallopian tubes, uterus, cervix, and superior vagina. Agenesis of the ducts naturally results in deficiencies in these structures; however, *müllerian agenesis* is a broad term that encompasses several different manifestations or classes. For example, class I patients lack a vagina and uterus but have normally functioning fallopian tubes and ovaries. Although the specific classes are beyond the scope of your exam, it will serve you well to note that variations may be presented.

Diagnostic Steps (Dx):

1. Pelvic ultrasound

Treatment and Management Steps (Tx/Mgmt):

1. Retroperitoneal ultrasound for additional abnormalities within the urinary or genital tract
2. Optional: surgical elongation of the vagina

Bicornuate Uterus, Uterine Didelphys

Buzz Words: Two uteri/cervixes/vaginas + dysmenorrhea + miscarriage + preterm labor + tampon not working

Clinical Presentation: A 24-year-old female with multiple miscarriages complains that her tampon does not adequately stop her menstrual flow. On pelvic exam, the patient is noted to have two uteri. She also complains of frequent urinary tract infections (UTIs).

PPx: N/A

MoD: Müllerian ducts fail to fuse in utero → two functional uteri, each leading to one ovary. The uterus, cervix, and upper vagina are formed by the fusion of the paramesonephric ducts in utero. Incomplete fusion may lead to a bicornuate uterus or uterine didelphys. A bicornuate uterus often manifests with a single vagina and cervix but a split or two-horned uterus. Further lack of fusion leads to uterine didelphys, which has two uteri, two cervixes, and possibly two vaginas. These are two distinguishable pathologies but they lie on the same spectrum, derived from the same pathology. Thus they are presented together.

Dx:
1. Transvaginal ultrasound or hysterosalpingogram (HSG).
2. Note: It is important to distinguish a bicornuate uterus from a septate uterus, as a septate uterus is associated with an increased risk of infertility.

Tx/Mgmt:
1. Uteroplasty/hysteroplasty/metroplasty if patient has recurrent miscarriages

Short Cervix/Cervical Insufficiency

Cervical insufficiency occurs when the cervix begins to dilate and efface before it is expected to, leading to preterm labor without normal contractions. The uterus is unable to retain the pregnancy.

Buzz Words: Recurrent second-trimester spontaneous abortions + no uterine contractions + bulging fetal membranes + bulging of amniotic sac to introitus + premature dilated cervix + <2.5 cm + prior loop electrocautery excision procedure (LEEP)/cone biopsy **+ funneling at the internal orifice of the uterus**

Clinical Presentation: Risk factors include LEEP, cone biopsy, and multiple gestations. Patients with a history of preterm birth, second-trimester pregnancy loss, prior obstetric trauma, or müllerian anomalies may also be predisposed to cervical insufficiency.

PPx: N/A

MoD: In utero developmental deficiency in tensile strength → cervical shortening early in pregnancy <2.5 cm at 20+ weeks' gestation → too weak to hold fetus through pregnancy → cervical dilation without uterine contractions → spontaneous abortion

Dx:

1. Cervical length measurement using transvaginal ultrasound

Tx/Mgmt:

1. Cervical cerclage to hold gestation through 38 weeks if the patient has history of preterm labor or recurrent spontaneous abortions

Neonatal Hydrocele

Buzz Words: Labial swelling + painless + canal of Nuck + inguinal canal

Clinical Presentation: An 8-month-old female presents with inguinolabial swelling.

PPx: N/A

MoD: Patent processus vaginalis or incomplete obliteration of canal of Nuck (parietal peritoneum pouch) → extends through inguinal canal to labia →

- Small hole → peritoneal fluid floods canal → hydrocele
- Large hole → bowel passes through canal → indirect inguinal hernia

Dx:

1. Ultrasound

Tx/Management:

1. Observation → spontaneous closure likely.
2. Surgical repair if infant suffers pain or hydrocele fails to resolve by age 2.

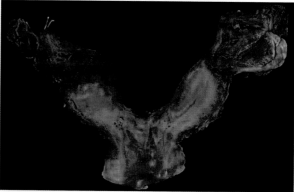

FIG. 11.1 Bicornate uterus. (https://en.wikipedia.org/wiki/Uterine_malformation#/media/File:Bicornuate_Uterus.jpg)

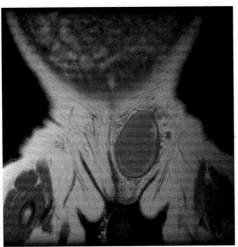

FIG. 11.2 Female neonate hydrocele. (From Park SJ, et al. Hydrocele of the canal of Nuck in a girl: ultrasound and MR appearance. Br J Radiol. 2004;77(915):243–244.)

GUNNER PRACTICE

1. A 29-year-old woman, G5P0, presents at 23 weeks' gestation for a prenatal visit. She has had no irregular bleeding, leakage, or pain. However, she is very nervous because she has had three unsuccessful pregnancies that have ended with spontaneous abortions around this time. On physical exam, her physician observes her to be 3.5-cm dilated. She is not experiencing contractions. What is the next best step in management?
   A. MRI
   B. Elective C-section
   C. Cervical cerclage
   D. Abort fetus immediately

2. A worried mother brings in her 3-month-old daughter, having noticed a large bulge in her groin. The infant has had cold symptoms for 2 days. Physical exam shows a golf-ball–sized, liquid-filled swelling on the right labial fold that can be transilluminated. What is the best step in management?
   A. Reassurance
   B. Emergency surgical repair
   C. Hernia reduction
   D. Ultrasound to check for incarcerated bowel
   E. Antibiotics

ANSWERS: What Would Gunner Jess/Jim Do?

1. WWGJD? A 29-year-old woman, G5P0, presents at 23 weeks for a prenatal visit. She has had no irregular bleeding, leakage, or pain. However, she is very nervous because she has had three unsuccessful pregnancies that have ended by spontaneous abortion around this time. On physical exam, her physicians observed her to be 3.5 cm dilated. She is not experiencing contractions. What is the next best step in management?

Answer: C. Cervical cerclage

Explanation: The patient most likely has cervical insufficiency, given her history of recurrent second-trimester miscarriages and spontaneous dilation. Her spontaneous dilation will lead to a spontaneous abortion; thus it must be prevented using cervical cerclage. This stitch adds support to the cervix, keeping the fetus in utero until 38 weeks, when the stitch can be removed.

A. MRI → Incorrect. MRI is not the proper imaging choice for cervical insufficiency.

B. Elective C-section → Incorrect. The baby is not yet viable and cannot be delivered now.

D. Abort fetus immediately → Incorrect. The patient is not at severe risk due to the pregnancy and can maintain a viable full gestation with the help of cervical cerclage.

2. WWGJD? A worried mother brings in her 3-month-old daughter after she noticed a large bulge in her groin. The infant has had cold symptoms for 2 days. Physical exam shows a golf-ball–sized, liquid-filled swelling on the right labial fold that can be transilluminated. What is the best step in management?

Answer: A. Reassurance

Explanation: This is a neonatal hydrocele filled with parietal peritoneal fluid. There is no evidence of incarcerated bowel in this patient, thus reassurance and observation is the best option. The hydrocele will most likely regress spontaneously.

B. Emergency surgical repair → Incorrect. Female neonatal hydroceles are not an emergent surgical issue.

C. Hernia reduction → Incorrect. Reduction may help with herniated bowel, but it will not reduce a hydrocele, as it is a fluid collection.

D. Ultrasound to check for incarcerated bowel →
    Incorrect. There is no evidence of incarcerated
    bowel in this patient that manifests as GI symptoms
    or a bulge that cannot be transilluminated.
E. Antibiotics → Incorrect. The labial bulge does not
    have an infectious etiology. The cold symptoms
    may be coincidental and do not require antibiotics.

12

Adverse Effects of Drugs on the Female Reproductive System

Kumar Nadhan, Hao-Hua Wu, and Leo Wang

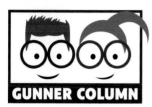

99 AR

Hormone replacement therapy overview

Introduction

There are many exogenous substances that may interfere with the normal function of the reproductive system and breasts. The substances most tested on the shelf exam are potent drugs like opioids and hormone replacement therapy (HRT). Notable others that are not commonly tested and therefore are not discussed in depth here are antihistamines, benzodiazepines, beta-blockers, and tricyclic antidepressants.

Medications Affecting the Female Reproductive System

Hormone Replacement Therapy

The subject of HRT and breast cancer has been controversial. Some studies suggest a causative link between HRT and breast cancer, others express a correlation, and some fail to show any association at all. The established diagnostic test for detecting early-stage breast cancer is mammography. Over time, breasts become less dense as the breast tissue is replaced by fat. HRT increases the density of breast tissue relative to the natural state. Breast cancer risk increases with age, so iatrogenically dense breasts may cloud mammographic interpretation and delay the diagnosis of an underlying malignancy.

Buzz Words: Breast tenderness + swollen/dense breasts + decreased sensitivity of mammography + postmenopausal + breast cancer

Clinical Presentation: A 54-year-old female on HRT for unbearable hot flashes presents with bilateral breast swelling and tenderness.

Prophylaxis (PPx): N/A

Mechanism of Disease (MoD): Estrogen → promotes breast growth

Diagnostic Steps (Dx):

1. Physical exam
2. Mammography

Treatment and Management Steps (Tx/Mgmt):

1. Continue HRT. Breast tenderness, swelling, and density are not contraindications for HRT.

Opioids

Although opioids provide relief for many patients who have tried other avenues of pain control, opioids also carry a high abuse potential. Opioids such as morphine and oxycodone exhibit an alarming trend toward addiction in the US population and are thus a hot topic for standardized exams. Opioids are most commonly prescribed for patients with chronic pain, and prolonged use by such patients may interfere with normal endocrine function.

Buzz Words: Depression + chronic pain + irregular menses + secondary amenorrhea

Clinical Presentation: A 41-year-old female on opioids for several years for her lower back pain presents with irregular menstrual cycles.

PPx: Alternative pain therapy

MoD: Hypogonadotropic hypogonadism: Prolonged opioid use → inhibits hypothalamic GnRH secretion → decreased LH and FSH→ decreased estradiol and progesterone

Dx:

1. Clinical presentation

Tx/Mgmt:

1. Rehabilitation
2. Alternative pain medication

Spironolactone

Spironolactone may be prescribed to help treat acne and hirsutism. Acne and hirsutism are frequently seen in patients with polycystic ovarian syndrome (PCOS). The side effects of spironolactone can include breast pain and irregular menses (although remember that one of the hallmarks of PCOS is infrequent menses or amenorrhea).

Buzz Words: Breast enlargement + breast pain + hypertension + hirsutism + acne + irregular menses + amenorrhea

Clinical Presentation: A 34-year-old female with severe acne and hirsutism, treated with spironolactone, presents with bilateral breast swelling and tenderness and an irregular menstrual cycle.

PPx: N/A

MoD: Unknown (see Gunner column)

Dx:

1. Clinical

Tx/Mgmt:

1. Discontinue spironolactone
2. Cycle estrogen/progesterone therapy along with spironolactone

QUICK TIPS

Spironolactone = gynecomastia in men = breast problems in women

Selective Serotonin Reuptake Inhibitors

Menstrual irregularities may result from prolonged use of selective serotonin reuptake inhibitors (SSRIs) or withdrawal from SSRIs. Mood changes and sexual side effects may result from SSRI use. SSRIs are also used to treat mood changes associated with the menstrual cycle, as in the case of premenstrual dysphoric disorder (PMDD).

Buzz Words: Breast pain + decreased libido + difficulty achieving orgasm + depression + panic disorder + obsessive compulsive disorder (OCD) + PMDD

Clinical Presentation: A 27-year-old female with a history of OCD and depression presents with difficulty achieving orgasm and decreased libido.

PPx: N/A

MoD: Unknown

Dx:

1. Clinical presentation

Tx/Mgmt:

1. Discontinue SSRI and switch to an alternate antidepressant

GUNNER PRACTICE

1. A 26-year-old woman comes into the office concerned that she may be pregnant. It has been 45 days since her last period. Her periods have been regular since menarche, with 28-day cycles. In the last 6 months, she has been experiencing heavy flow and severe cramping, for which she takes an extra dose of her chronic pain medication. Serum beta-HCG test is negative. She currently complains of no other symptoms. The patient was recently diagnosed with type 2 diabetes mellitus, for which she is taking metformin, but she says that she fails to take it regularly. She has a family history of breast cancer and has two children at home. What is the most likely cause of her irregular menses?

   A. Pregnancy
   B. HPA axis dysfunction
   C. Turner syndrome
   D. Thyroid disease
   E. Diabetes

2. A 55-year-old woman visits the clinic for a screening mammogram. She states that she examines herself often and has not found any areas that worry her. She has a family history of breast cancer involving her mother and aunt. She had her last menstrual cycle 4

years earlier. She has had severe hot flashes and vaginal dryness, for which she started a hormone medication. What are the most likely findings on mammography?

A. Ductal carcinoma in situ
B. Fibrocystic breast disease
C. Invasive ductal carcinoma
D. Decreased fatty tissue compared with premenopause
E. Absent ductal and glandular tissue

ANSWERS: What Would Gunner Jess/Jim Do?

1. WWGJD? A 26-year-old woman comes into the office concerned that she may be pregnant. It has been 45 days since her last period. Her period has been regular since menarche, with 28 day cycles. In the last 6 months, she has been experiencing heavy flow and severe cramping for which she takes an extra dose of her chronic pain medication. Serum beta-hCG test is negative. She currently complains of no other symptoms. The patient was recently diagnosed with type 2 diabetes mellitus, for which she is prescribed metformin, but says she fails to take it regularly. She has a family history of breast cancer and has two children at home. What is the most likely cause of her irregular menses?

Answer: B. HPA axis dysfunction

> Explanation: The patient most likely is experiencing irregular menses from opioid abuse. She states she uses chronic pain medication. Opioids may cause menstrual irregularity through hypogonadotropic hypogonadism.
>
> A.   Pregnancy→ Incorrect. The patient has a negative serum hCG so is most likely not pregnant.
>
> C.   Turner syndrome → Incorrect. Turner would be diagnosed at an earlier age, presenting with primary amenorrhea. The patient has had regular menstrual cycles and has given birth to two children, both contradictory to a diagnosis of Turner.
>
> D.   Thyroid disease → Incorrect. Although thyroid disease is a common cause of irregular menses, the patient exhibits no signs of thyroid dysfunction.
>
> E.   Diabetes → Incorrect. Uncontrolled diabetes may affect menstruation; however, this is not common. The patient was only recently diagnosed with diabetes. The chances are low that it has become extreme enough to affect menstruation.

2. WWGJD? A 55-year-old woman visits the clinic for a breast screening mammogram. The patient states that she examines herself often and has not found any areas that worry her. She has a family history of breast cancer in her mother and aunt. She had her last menstrual cycle 4 years ago. She has had severe hot flashes and vaginal dryness, for which she started a hormone medication. What are the most likely findings on mammography?

Answer: B. Fibrocystic breast disease

Explanation: HRT stimulates growth of fibrous tissue in the breast, which can make the breast feel lumpy. On mammography, the breast appears dense.

A. Ductal carcinoma in situ → Incorrect. Cancer is not suspected in this patient despite the family history.

C. Invasive ductal carcinoma → Incorrect. Malignancy is not suspected in this patient.

D. Decreased fatty tissue compared with premenopause → Incorrect. Fatty tissue increases in breasts with age, especially after menopause. The HRT will reduce the amount of tissue replaced by fatty tissue, but there will still be more fat than before menopause.

E. Absent ductal and glandular tissue → Incorrect. Ductal and glandular tissue decrease after menopause but will not be absent in the breast. HRT will preserve this tissue relative to postmenopausal patients without hormone replacement.

Prenatal Care

Leo Wang, Hao-Hua Wu, Rebecca W. Gao,
and Cynthia DeTata

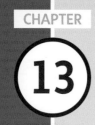

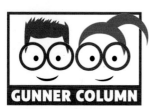
Introduction

This chapter focuses on prophylactic measures to support women as they make decisions to get pregnant, carry a pregnancy, and deliver a baby.

Preconception Counseling and Care

Preconception care is preventive risk identification and management in order to maximize the chances of a healthy pregnancy for the mother and fetus. Nutritional counseling is important, as well as making sure that vaccinations are up to date. Identification of health issues and medicines that are contraindicated in pregnancy is crucial to prevent problems. Organogenesis in the fetus occurs before 9 weeks. Most women present for obstetric care after the period of organogenesis is complete. Caring for a woman of reproductive age involves counseling regarding the risks of carrying a pregnancy due to medical problems as well as the risk to the fetus from medications. It is preferable to treat women of reproductive age with medicines that are not teratogenic. Patients also need to know that discontinuing some medications such as hypoglycemics and thyroid hormones can put the fetus at risk. Hyperglycemia can cause fetal malformations or pregnancy loss. Hypothyroidism can affect fetal brain development. Pregnancy can become life threatening to women with certain medical conditions. They may not know this until they are pregnant and need to consider either terminating or continuing the pregnancy.

Nutritional Assessment

An unhealthy weight or poor nutrition can affect both maternal and fetal well-being during pregnancy. Overweight or obese women have an increased risk of preeclampsia or gestational diabetes, operative delivery, birth defects, preterm delivery, and fetal demise. Underweight women are at increased risk of preterm labor, preterm delivery, and poor fetal growth. Folate supplementation is a critical aspect of prenatal care to prevent neural tube defects.

Prophylaxis (PPx): Weight is a modifiable risk factor, best dealt with prior to pregnancy.

Mechanism of Disease (MoD): Obesity → insulin resistance → gestational diabetes mellitus (GDM)

Diagnostic Steps (Dx):

1. Assess the ABCDs of nutrition, see Table 13.1:
   - Anthropometric factors (weight, height, etc.)
   - Biochemical factors (anemia) via complete blood count (CBC), basic metabolic panel (BMP)
   - Clinical factors (lifestyle)
   - Dietary risks
2. Woman's understanding of pregnancy and complications that may occur secondary to any medical illness she may have

Treatment and Management Steps (Tx/Mgmt):

1. Dietary and lifestyle modifications

Rh Screening

Red blood cells (RBCs) are screened for AB and Rh type. Eighty-five percent of Caucasians, 95% of African-Americans, and 99% of Asians are Rh-positive. If an Rh-negative woman procreates with an Rh-positive man, the fetus may be Rh-positive. Maternal exposure to the fetus's Rh-positive antigens can lead to the development of maternal antibodies against the Rh protein. If a future fetus is then Rh-positive, the maternal immune system will identify the Rh-positive fetal cells as foreign, leading to fetal RBC hemolysis, severe anemia, hydrops, or fetal death. To prevent Rh-isoimmunization, Rh-negative women are given Rho(D) immune globulin (RhoGAM), injected at 28 weeks and at delivery if the newborn is Rh-positive. Rho(D) immune globulin is also given whenever there is the potential for mixing of fetal and maternal blood (e.g., miscarriage, chorionic villous sampling, amniocentesis, abdominal trauma, version).

PPx: Test women for their Rh status and give Rh-negative women Rho(D) immune globulin as indicated earlier. If a woman has already had a previous pregnancy, test for Rh antibodies. Once a woman is Rh antibody–positive, giving Rho(D) immune globulin is not helpful. A woman suspected of being Rh antibody–positive should be counseled regarding the severe risks to her fetus. If she chooses to continue the pregnancy, she should be followed by a high-risk obstetrician with serial antibody titers and ultrasounds.

MoD: If an Rh-negative woman is exposed to Rh antigens from an Rh-positive fetus, she will form antibodies that

TABLE 13.1 Nutritional Needs During Preconception and Pregnancy

	Preconception	Pregnancy
Calories	Calories to attain healthy weight prior to pregnancy	2100 calories/day; <14 y/o may require 2300/day, obese patients need individualized dietary plans
Proteins	0.8 g/kg per day	1st half: 0.8 g/kg per day 2nd half: 1.1 g/kg per day
Carbohydrates	Individualized	175 g/d unless diabetic, where there should be carb restriction
Fat	<10% calories from sat fats, poly-unsaturated fat ~10%, rest of fat intake = monounsaturated fat	<10% calories from sat fats, poly-unsaturated fat ~10%, rest of fat intake = monounsaturated fat
Nonnutritive sweeteners	Acesulfame potassium, aspartame, saccharin, sucralose, neotame are all acceptable	Acesulfame potassium, aspartame, saccharin, sucralose, neotame are all acceptable
Fiber	25 g/d	28 g/d
Sodium	1.5 g/d	<2.3 g/d
Folic acid	**400 µg/d:** Women with prior fetus with neural tube defect should take 4 mg/d	600–800 µg/d for 14–18 y/o; 600–1000 µg/d for >19 years
Iron	18 mg/d	27 mg/d
Calcium	1300 mg/d for 14–18 y/o; 1000 mg/d for 19+ y/o	1300 mg/d for 14–18 y/o; 1000 mg/d for 19+ y/o
Multivitamin supplementation	Only if evidence of undernutrition	Recommended for all women; avoid oversupplementation of vitamin A and D; 4000 IU vit D daily
Caffeine	>500 mg/day can delay conception	Do not exceed >300 mg/day (poor evidence)
Alcohol	Avoid as can decrease fertility	**NO**
Smoking	Cessation	**NO**

will complicate future pregnancies. Rho(D) immune globulin binds any fetal blood Rh in the maternal circulation, thereby preventing the maternal immune system from recognizing it and mounting a response.

Dx:

1. Blood test for Rh factor

Tx/Mgmt:

1. Intramuscular (IM)/intravenous (IV) administration of Rho(D) immune globulin for prophylaxis.
2. If a woman has been sensitized, is pregnant, and chooses to continue her pregnancy despite the risks to the fetus, she should be followed with serial antibody titers and ultrasounds.
3. If developing hydrops, the fetus can be treated with an intrauterine transfusion or early delivery.

Immunizations and Screenings

All women should be immunized against **hepatitis B, influenza, rubella** (measles, mumps, rubella [MMR] vaccine), **pertussis** (tetanus, diphtheria, pertussis [TDAP] vaccine), and **varicella**. Rubella and varicella vaccines cannot be given during pregnancy since they are live-virus vaccines. Shingles is not dangerous to the fetus and vaccinating and treating the mother with antiretrovirals are both safe. Women should also have Pap screening for cervical cancer as per American Society for Colposcopy and Cervical Pathology (ASCCP) guidelines.

Screening for Alpha-Fetoprotein/Neural Tube Defect

PPx: Alpha-fetoprotein (AFP) level testing is offered to all women. It is done between the 14th and 22nd weeks of pregnancy, typically as part of a maternal serum triple or quadruple screening test (it also includes human chorionic gonadotropin [hCG], unconjugated estriol estrogen, and inhibin A). AFP is found in fetal serum and amniotic fluid and is made early from fetal yolk sac and later in the liver and gastrointestinal (GI) tract.
- High levels of AFP → spina bifida or other neural tube defects, anencephaly
- Low AFP → Down syndrome, Edwards syndrome

Other Assessments

Here are few key additional recommendations for women of childbearing age who plan to become pregnant:
- Diabetes = good glycemic control and dietary counseling
- Hypothyroidism = appropriate levothyroxine dosing
- Phenylketonuria (PKU) = proper dietary restrictions
- Warfarin therapy = switch to a different anticoagulant
  - Early exposure to warfarin → **coumarin embryopathy**: facial abnormalities, optic atrophy, digital abnormalities, mental impairment, fetal bleeding
  - Later exposure → central nervous system (CNS) defects
  - High-risk situations (mechanical heart valve) should involve education regarding the increased risk of thromboembolism during pregnancy and the risk of fetal embryopathy. Ideally these patients should be counseled about risks prior to conception and offered contraception. Patients may choose to terminate the pregnancy. Changing to low-molecular-weight heparin (LMWH) treatment is warranted to avoid coumarin embryopathy. No matter which anticoagulant is used, the patient is at increased risk of thromboembolism.

- **LMWHs** are easiest to use during pregnancy, and most patients requiring anticoagulation should consider being switched to LMWH during the preconception period. Patients on LMWH should be switched to heparin near delivery so as to decrease the risk of hemorrhage.
- Antiepileptics = NO antiepileptic drug has been proven to be safe. Considering lowering dosage or tapering off.
  - Avoid **valproic acid** (neural tube defects and spina bifida, atrioseptal defect, craniosyostosis, polydactyly, hypospadias)
  - Newer antiepileptic drugs have a 1%–2% risk of anomalies.
- Isotretinoin for skin conditions (e.g., acne) = patients should be on reliable contraception and should **not** get pregnant until 6 months after cessation of isotretinoin usage. Men and women prescribed isotretinoin must register for a national database known as iPLEDGE indicating that they are aware of the teratogenic effects (e.g., severe mental deficits, facial and cardiac abnormalities) in order to use the medication.

Adolescent Pregnancy and Preventing Complications of Adolescent Pregnancies

Buzz Words: Pregnancy in women aged 13–19

Clinical Presentation: Ages 13–19 are considered adolescent pregnancies; they are at increased risk of preterm delivery, low birth weight, and infant mortality. Teenage mothers are also less likely to graduate from high school or to have the resources needed for raising a child. They are more likely to live in poverty, to be victims of abuse and neglect themselves, and to neglect their newborn.

PPx: Encourage effective contraception. Discuss pregnancy risks frequently.

MoD: Young maternal age can lead to physical complications and also increases risks of social and mental complications such as emotional, physical, or sexual abuse, partner violence, and risky behaviors.

Dx: N/A

Tx/Mgmt:

1. Adequate counseling and education regarding healthy pregnancy, breastfeeding, infant care, and postpartum contraception
2. Social development programs, referral for assistance in completing high school
3. Child Protective Services (CPS) reporting according to minor consent laws, screen for incest, sex trafficking

Prenatal Risk Assessment/Prevention

Prenatal risk assessment and prevention includes identification of factors or illnesses that could put the health of the mother or fetus at risk, with education or treatment as needed.

Antepartum Fetal Evaluation

The goal of antepartum fetal evaluation is to **prevent fetal ischemic encephalopathy and fetal demise.** However, antepartum fetal evaluation **has not been definitively demonstrated to improve neonatal outcome via randomized controlled studies.** There is circumstantial evidence that monitoring improves outcome as compared with pregnancies that are unmonitored (and presumably at lower risk). Various monitoring techniques are used in situations where the risks of fetal death or growth complications are high. Initiation of testing should occur between weeks 32 and 34; in particularly severe cases, testing may begin as early as week 26. The following summarizes the American College of Obstetricians and Gynecologists (ACOG) guidelines on antepartum fetal surveillance and the various uses of different screening techniques in order of least to most invasive.

Fetal Movement Assessment

All pregnant women are asked to monitor fetal movements. After 28 weeks, the mother should be able to count 10 movements within 30 minutes at least once a day. If the mother notes decreased or absent movement, additional testing is warranted.

Nonstress Test

The fetal heart rate is monitored externally for 20 minutes. Two accelerations 15 beats above baseline lasting 15 seconds is considered reactive and indicates a nonacidotic, well-oxygenated fetus.

Biophysical Profile

The biophysical profile is the nonstress test in combination with ultrasound testing. In addition to nonstress testing, components from ultrasound include the presence of fetal breathing movements, fetal limb movements, fetal limb tone, and amniotic fluid volume. Each of the five components, if normal, receives a score of 2, and a total score of 8–10 is normal. A score of 6–8 warrants repeat testing in 24 hours and a score of less than 4 warrants delivery, although decision making should be individualized if the fetus is preterm.

Amniotic fluid is made both by placental transudate and fetal urine, a normal index of 8–20 is reassuring. Between 5 and 8 is borderline and the test should be repeated after hydration. Less than 5 is oligohydramnios and warrants delivery if the fetus is near term or intensive monitoring, steroids, and plan for delivery if the fetus is preterm. Greater than 20 is polyhydramnios and can be associated with uncontrolled diabetes, fetal anomalies, hydrops, or idiopathic poor outcome.

Umbilical Artery Doppler Velocimetry

Measurement of diastolic flow in the umbilical artery. High-velocity diastolic flow is normal, whereas low-velocity flow is of concern in the setting of **intrauterine growth restriction**. In severe cases, the flow can be reversed.

Contraction Stress Test

Tests response of fetal heart rate to uterine contractions. Late decelerations in heart rate are associated possible fetal hypoxia, poor placental perfusion, or fetal compromise. Left untreated, this can lead to growth restriction, neonatal encephalopathy, or fetal death (Fig. 13.1). There are four potential results:

- Negative: No late decelerations
- Positive: Late decelerations after >50% of contractions
- Equivocal-suspicious: Intermittent late decelerations or variable decelerations
- Equivocal-hyperstimulatory: Fetal heart rate decelerations in the presence of contractions that occur once every 2 minutes or last >90 seconds
- Unsatisfactory: <3 contractions in 10 minutes → cannot interpret

Genetic Screening of Newborns

A newborn screening panel tests for many disorders, but **this varies from state to state**. Physicians should recognize the newborn screening panel in their particular states. The three diseases that are screened for in **all** states are congenital hypothyroidism, galactosemia, and phenylketonuria. Other high-yield diseases to know include congenital adrenal hyperplasia, sickle cell disease, congenital heart disease, cystic fibrosis, severe combined immune deficiency (SCID), maple syrup urine disease, and Pompe disease.

A blood spot specimen obtained as close to hospital discharge as possible should be used for screening. An important point is to **ensure adequate communication of results**. Important follow-up is of utmost priority, especially in the presence of a positive test result.

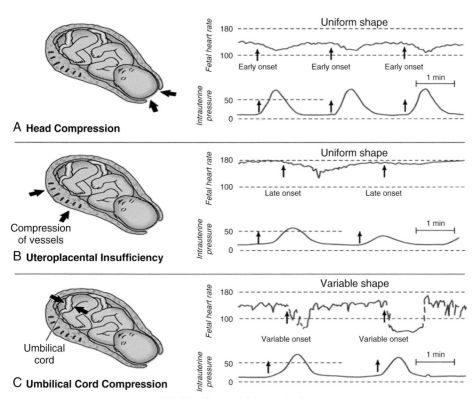

FIG. 13.1 Abnormal fetal monitoring.

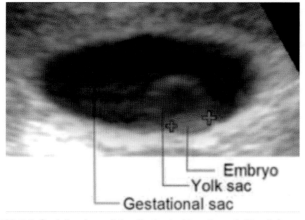

FIG. 13.2 Gestational sac. (https://upload.wikimedia.org/wikipedia/commons/0/06/Ultrasound_of_embryo_at_5_weeks%2C_colored.png).

Neonatal Diabetes Screening

Neonatal diabetes can lead to neurologic problems and epilepsy; it is characterized by hyperglycemia after birth and is often inherited in an autosomal dominant fashion. This disease will present within the first 6 months of life.

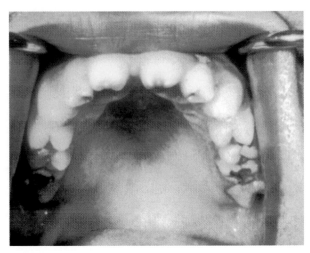

FIG. 13.3 Hutchinson teeth. (https://upload.wikimedia.org/wikipedia/commons/9/96/Hutchinson_teeth_congenital_syphilis_PHIL_2385.rsh.jpg).

All babies <6 months of age with hyperglycemia should receive genetic testing for monogenic inherited forms of diabetes.

Supervision of Normal Pregnancy

Assessment of Gestational Age

By convention, a pregnancy lasts 40 weeks, as measured from the first day of the LMP. The estimated due date is calculated by both menstrual period dating and ultrasound confirmation of dating. Gestational age is the age of fetus based on the calculated due date. In the newborn, calculated gestational age is determined from physical exam and the Ballard score.

Prenatal Dating

From physical exam:

Uterine size: Uterus compared to fruit: 6- to 8-week size = plum, 8- to 10-week size = orange, 10- to 12-week size = grapefruit. After 12 weeks, the uterus can be palpated above the pubic symphysis. At 16 weeks, the uterine fundus can be palpated between the pubic symphysis and the umbilicus. By 20 weeks, the uterine fundus can be palpated at the umbilicus. After 20 weeks, the fundus should be 1 cm above the umbilicus for each week of gestation (e.g., 30 weeks' gestation = 30 cm from the pubic symphysis to the fundus).

Naegele's rule → estimated date of delivery: Add 1 year + 3 months to LMP, subtract 1 week.

From ultrasound:
- The earliest ultrasound is the best, as the error of measurement increases with gestational age:
  - First trimester ± 1 week
  - Second trimester ± 2 weeks
  - Third trimester ± 3 weeks
- Use the LMP for gestational age calculation unless there is an ultrasound discrepancy. If the difference between LMP and gestational age as measured on ultrasound is greater than the error of measurement, the ultrasound is used, otherwise the LMP is used.
- Yolk sac should appear at 5 weeks and degrade by 12 weeks, but is a poor predictor of gestational age.
- Crown–rump length: Straight-line measurement of length of embryo. At 7–10 weeks, this is the most accurate measure of gestational age.

Postnatal Dating
- Dubowitz: 13 physical and neurologic assessments, higher scores → greater maturity
  - Bad in preterm infants
- Ballard score: 12 physical and neurologic assessments, performed at 30–42 hours of age (easier to perform than Dubowitz but not as accurate)
- New Ballard score: For preterm babies
- Eye examination: Disappearance of anterior vascular capsule → 27–34 weeks gestation, used for rapid assessment
- Electroencephalography (EEG): Characteristic EEG pattern beginning at 21–22 weeks

Iron-Deficiency Anemia and Prevention

Buzz Words: Shortness of breath + dizziness + headaches + pallor + fatigue + pica + spoon-shaped nails

Clinical Presentation: Pregnancy elevates the risk of iron-deficiency anemia, which can manifest with a microcytic anemia and any of the features presented in the buzz words section. **Prevent** iron-deficiency anemia in pregnancy with an adequate diet high in iron and supplementation as needed. Women who have had multiple pregnancies are at increased risk of anemia, which can worsen rapidly with postpartum blood loss. Women with anemia suffer fatigue and are at increased risk of postpartum depression. The fetus may be at risk of growth restriction.

PPx: Vitamin C + iron diet, particular care in gastric bypass patients (should have coated supplements absorbed in intestine rather than stomach)

MoD: Iron required for heme synthesis. Vitamin C improves iron reabsorption.

Dx:
1. In first and third trimesters, Hct and Hbg <33% and <11 g/dL → anemia
2. In second trimester, <32% and <10.5 g/dL → anemia
3. Differentiate between iron-deficiency anemia and anemia caused by deficiency of vitamin B12 and folate (megaloblastic) or hemoglobinopathies such as thalassemia or sickle cell disease

Tx/Mgmt:
1. Iron supplementation

Weight Management and Nutrition

Normal weight gain: 25–35 pounds, additional 300 calories per day. A gain of 4–6 pounds in the first trimester and 1 pound a week in the second and third trimesters is normal. Underweight women should gain up to 40 pounds. Overweight women should gain 10–15 pounds. Exceeding recommended weight gain increases risk of gestational diabetes, macrosomia, and difficulty with delivery as well as hypertensive disorders of pregnancy and preeclampsia. Obesity can be associated with increased risk of operative delivery, fetal growth problems, and unexplained fetal demise.

Gaining too much increases risk of musculoskeletal complaints such as backaches and varicose veins; it also makes postpartum weight loss more difficult.

Ensure adequate folic acid and vitamins in diet.

Maternal, Fetal, and Newborn Infections

99 AR

TORCH maternal-fetal infections overview and images

The following infections are either screened for, prevented, or treated. Transmission of infection to the fetus can lead to pregnancy loss, intrauterine fetal death (IUFD), deformity, delay of developmental milestones, or congenital infections otherwise affecting the health of the child after delivery.

Cytomegalovirus (CMV)

99 AR

Neonatal CMV infections

Buzz Words: Periventricular calcifications + premature birth + small head + seizures + petechial rash + hepatosplenomegaly + jaundice

PPx: Most people are exposed as children and are already immune. There is no treatment for infection in the mother, as most infection is unrecognized. Avoid infection by handwashing.

MoD: If the mother is infected, the highest rate of transmission is in the third trimester, but it is most severe in first trimester.

Dx:
1. IgG/IgM in blood
2. Polymerase chain reaction (PCR) of amniotic fluid

Tx/Mgmt:
1. Ganciclovir and valcyclovir

Hepatitis B

Buzz Words: Jaundice + dark urine + nausea/vomiting + maternal IV drug use + chronic carriers

PPx: Screen all mothers for active hepatitis B. Most pregnant patients are asymptomatic chronic carriers.

MoD: HBV transmission through blood, semen, vaginal secretion, saliva to the mother, through exposure at delivery.

Dx:
1. Hepatitis B PCR, Hep B antigen, viral load

Tx/Mgmt:
1. The risk of fetal infection is highest if the mother contracts Hep B in the third trimester—give women at risk Hep B vaccination during pregnancy.
2. If a woman is exposed during pregnancy, give Hep B immunoglobulin (HBIG) as soon as possible and vaccinate:
   - If mother is **negative** for active hepatitis B, give HBV vaccine to baby after birth. Routine vaccination schedule may be delayed up to 2 months of age.
   - If mother is **positive** for active hepatitis B, check liver function and viral load. Antiviral treatment may be needed. Vaccinate patient and partner against Hep A, partner against Hep B. During delivery, reduce exposure by avoiding fetal scalp electrode (FSC) or scalp sampling. The newborn should have HBIG (Hep B immunoglobulin) and the Hep B vaccination at birth. There is no contraindication to breastfeeding.

Rubella

Buzz Words: Deafness + eye abnormalities (e.g., cataracts) + congenital heart disease (TRIAD) + thrombocytopenic purpura

Clinical Presentation: Other presenting features include spleen/liver problems, intellectual disability, microcephaly, micrognathia, low birth weight. Baby should also be assessed for development of mental or psychiatric disorders. Many infants with congenital rubella appear normal at birth but later develop complications.

PPx: MMR vaccine prior to conception (CANNOT be given during pregnancy since it is a live-virus vaccine). Testing for rubella immunity is part of routine prenatal care, if

99 AR

Pediatric mnemonics

nonimmune, patient should be given MMR prior to leaving the hospital postpartum.

MoD: Contraction of rubella during first trimester—risk of spontaneous abortion (SAB) and congenital rubella syndrome. Transmission 80% in first trimester, 25% in second and third trimester.

Tx/Mgmt:
1. Vaccinate prior to pregnancy.
2. Mothers who are rubella nonimmune should avoid sick children with rash and wash hands frequently.
3. Alert pediatricians regarding risk of infection.

Herpes Simplex Virus (HSV)/Neonatal HSV

Buzz Words: Vesicular lesions on skin, eye, mouth + herpes in mother (vesicles on vagina)

PPx: History of prior outbreaks, physical exam, STD counseling

MoD: Vertical transmission of HSV (type 2 mostly) from mother to baby via direct contact with lesions at delivery

Dx:
1. Clinical presentation/ prior history maternal herpes

Tx/Mgmt:
1. Acyclovir suppression starting at 36 weeks to reduce risk of outbreak
2. If active herpes infection, deliver via C-section

Human Immunodeficiency Virus

Buzz Words: Enlarged lymph nodes + immunosuppression in baby + failure to thrive

Clinical Presentation: Human immunodeficiency virus (HIV) from physical exam will present as candidiasis, oral thrush, oral leukoplakia, parotid enlargement with aphthous ulcers, HIV dermatitis. Most mothers with positive HIV found in prenatal care are asymptomatic and unaware of the disease.

PPx: Treatment in symptomatic mothers depends on symptoms and viral load. In asymptomatic women, zidovudine reduces transmission to baby—from as much at 25% down to 8%.

MoD: Vertical transmission of HIV during pregnancy or delivery. Can also be passed on via breast milk.

Dx:
1. HIV antibody, viral load testing

Tx/Mgmt:
1. Treatment of symptomatic mothers as necessary
2. Zidovudine to reduce transmission during birth. Treatment to reduce viral load to undetectable levels and avoiding exposure during delivery can reduce transmission rate from 25%–1%.

3. Vaginal delivery versus C-section depending on viral load. Exposure during delivery can be reduced by planned cesarean prior to rupture of membranes. With an undetectable viral load, women can labor but use of FSE, scalp sampling, vacuum, or forceps must be avoided.

Influenza

Buzz Words: Lack of vaccinations + sniffling + runny nose/congestion + sneezing + sore throat + winter + muscle ache/fatigue **+ high fever** + chest tightness

Clinical Presentation: "The flu" is caused by the influenza virus. Differentiate a cold from influenza by the presence of a **high fever, GI symptoms** → **testing.** The Centers for Disease Control (CDC) recommend that all pregnant patients **receive the influenza vaccine.** During pregnancy, influenza can progress to a severe life-threatening illness in the mother. Severe illness from the flu can lead to preterm labor.

PPx: Frequent handwashing + annual influenza vaccine

MoD: Respiratory droplet transmission of influenza A, B, or C. Influenza A is most common and includes the H1N1–H7N9 viruses. Viruses bind to **hemagluttinin** on epithelial cells → replication. **Neuraminidase** leads to release of viral particles from host cells.

Dx:
1. Clinical suspicion
2. Rapid influenza test of pregnant patients suspected to have the flu as they can become very ill
3. Other tests exist (PCR, antigen detection, viral culture) but are used only when absolutely critical to make influenza diagnosis (as in health care worker, etc.).

Tx/Mgmt:
1. Acetaminophen/hydration, (avoid NSAIDs in pregnancy)
2. Oseltamivir, zanamivir, peramivir are all approved for pregnant women
3. Influenza vaccine should be offered and encouraged for all pregnant women.

Parvovirus B19

Buzz Words: Baby with severe anemia + "slapped cheek" rash in pregnant woman

Clinical Presentation: Fifth disease is not a common infection in pregnant women, as most are immune due to childhood exposure. Consider testing pregnant preschool teachers for immunity or others who work with young children. Avoid exposure by washing hands and staying away from ill children with rash. If maternal infection occurs, particularly in the first trimester, the virus can attack and lyse fetal blood cells, leading to severe anemia, hydrops, and fetal demise.

PPx: Oral/respiratory hygiene

MoD: Parvovirus B19 infection from respiratory droplets

Dx:

1. Clinical, though lab tests are available.

Tx/Mgmt:

1. Supportive

Varicella Zoster Virus (VZV)

Buzz Words: Fever, malaise, painful skin rash in mother with skin lesions in newborn + microcephaly + limb hypoplasia + cataracts

Clinical Presentation: Primary infection of VZV in mother during the first trimester of pregnancy can lead to congenital varicella syndrome. This presents with skin lesions, ocular defects (cataracts, chorioretinitis, Horner, nystagmus), limb abnormalities, microcephaly, CNS abnormalities (seizures), and mental delay.

PPx:

- Vaccinate women before pregnancy, cannot vaccinate during pregnancy as this is a live-virus vaccine.
- If exposed during pregnancy, varicella immunoglobulin (VZIG) or acyclovir for 5–7 days can reduce the possibility of infection.

MoD: Hematogenous dissemination of virus can affect newborn.

Dx:

1. Clinical/PCR lab testing

Tx/Mgmt:

1. Admit to hospital and give IV acyclovir to mother if she is actively infected. Varicella infection can be more severe and can progress to pneumonia in pregnancy.
2. If the mother is infected within 5–7 days of delivery → neonatal infection may ensue. This can be severe, leading to neonatal death. Alert pediatricians.

Chlamydia trachomatis (Neonatal Chlamydia)

Buzz words: Conjunctivitis + pneumonia + afebrile newborn

PPx: All pregnant women are screened for asymptomatic chlamydial infection. Patient and partner are treated, and a test of cure is done to ensure complete treatment.

MoD: Active transmission of *Chlamydia*

Dx:

1. PCR testing of endocervical or urine sample at the beginning of pregnancy; rescreen if STD exposure suspected during pregnancy.

99 AR

Neonatal conjunctivitis

Tx/Mgmt:
1. Treatment of patient and partner during pregnancy, with test of cure.
2. Erythromycin eye ointment is given routinely to all newborns in case of recent asymptomatic infection.

Treponema pallidum (Congenital Syphilis)

Clinical Presentation: Most often asymptomatic latent syphilis in the mother. Complications can lead to blindness, deafness, deformity.

PPx: FTA-ABS/RPR/VDRL in pregnant woman, treat latent and active syphilis with penicillin (PCN) in order to avoid transmission through the placenta during pregnancy to the fetus and to avoid transmission through the meninges, causing tertiary syphilis.

MoD: Transmission during pregnancy through the placenta. Vertical transmission from mom to baby.

Dx:
1. Positive RPR or other screening with confirmatory testing and titer

Tx/Mgmt:
1. PCN—There are no good substitutes for PCN.
   - PCN passes through the placenta to treat the fetus.
   - If a patient is PCN-allergic, she is admitted to the intensive care unit (ICU) for desensitization in order to treat.
   - Posttreatment titers should be followed; retreat if rising.

Group B Strep (GBS)

Buzz Words: Vomiting and irritability, meningitis, pneumonia in the newborn

99 AR

Neonatal Group B strep screening and infection, CDC

Clinical Presentation: GBS is part of normal vaginal flora in 20%–40% of pregnant women. It is asymptomatic but can cause early- or late-onset infection in the newborn and postpartum endometritis.

PPx:
   - Identify GBS-positive women by lower vaginal and rectal cultures from weeks 35–37.
   - If a patient has a GBS-positive urine culture, she is also considered to be colonized with GBS.
   - GBS-positive women should receive IV PCN or ampicillin >4 hours before delivery.

MoD: Transmission during birth. Ascension of GBS bacteria into the uterus after rupture of membranes

Dx:
1. Lower vaginal and rectal culture (must be done prior to delivery as not enough time if woman presents in labor).

2. Check sensitivities with culture if patient is allergic to PCN.
3. If less than 37 weeks and GBS status unknown → treat with antibiotics.

Tx/Mgmt:
1. PCN

Toxoplasma gondii–Toxoplasmosis

Buzz Words: Raw meat + cat litter + mental retardation + chorioretinitis

Clinical Presentation: Infection from ingestion of parasitic cysts in undercooked or raw meat or from exposure to cat feces, most often asymptomatic. Infection may be undetected until newborn has signs of severe mental retardation, chorioretinitis, blindness, epilepsy, intracranial calcifications, and hydrocephalus. May cause fetal loss during pregnancy.

PPx: Most adults are immune from prior exposure. If not immune, exposure leading to maternal infection may be asymptomatic.
- Pregnant women should avoid undercooked meat and changing cat litter.
- If infection suspected:
    - Amniotic fluid PCR after 18 weeks' gestation
    - Tx infection with spiramycin in mother

MoD: Parasite can pass through placenta, infecting fetus.

Dx:
1. Serologic tests and PCR in newborn suspected to have congenital toxoplasmosis

Tx/Mgmt:
1. Tx infection with spiramycin in mother, followed by treatment of newborn by pediatricians.

Amnionitis/Chorioamnionitis

Buzz Words: Fetal tachycardia

Clinical Presentation: A patient can have amnionitis with or without contractions, but an ill patient with chorioamnionitis might present with preterm contractions if ill, flu-like symptoms and fever, tender uterus, prolonged labor, and/or prolonged rupture of amniotic membranes + association with cerebral palsy.

MoD: Inflammation of fetal membranes, bacteria ascending from vagina into uterus

Dx:
1. Maternal fever + WBCs >15,000 or HR > 100 or fetal heart rate (FHR) >160 or uterine tenderness or foul odor of amniotic fluid, fetal or maternal tachycardia

Tx/Mgmt:
1. Ampicillin + gentamicin. Add clindamycin after delivery.

gg AR

Chorioamnionitis ACOG clinical guidelines

Urinary Tract Infection

Urinary tract infection (UTI) risk is increased in pregnancy due to anatomic changes to the urinary tract caused by the enlarging uterus. UTIs in pregnant women are considered "complicated UTIs" and should have culture and sensitivities as part of testing as well as a follow-up test of cure. Antibiotics that can be safely used in pregnancy include PCNs, cephalosporins, and erythromycin.

Screening for asymptomatic bacteriuria is part of prenatal care. Asymptomatic bacteriuria can progress to pyelonephritis and severe illness; it can trigger preterm labor and thus should be treated. A follow-up culture should be done as a test of cure.

GUNNER PRACTICE

1. A 32-year-old gravida 2 para 1 woman at 34 weeks' gestation comes in for a prenatal checkup. She had an appointment a week earlier but canceled because of a family emergency. She appears tired but states that she is otherwise fine. She denies vaginal bleeding, contractions, or fluid leakage. She is still able to feel her baby kick throughout the day. Her only medications right now are folate supplements and metformin. She had cut down her cigarette use but recently began smoking a pack a day because of the family emergency. She denies the use of alcohol or other substances. Vitals are 110/70 mm Hg, 90 bpm, 98.6 °F, 20 RR. Physical exam is within normal limits for gestational age. On exam, fetal heart sounds are appreciable on Doppler. What is the next best step in management?
   A. Quad screen
   B. Amniocentesis
   C. Pregnancy-associated plasma protein A and beta-hCG
   D. Biophysical profile
   E. Fetal fibronectin test

ANSWER: What Would Gunner Jess/Jim Do?

1. WWGJD? A 32-year-old, gravida 2, para 1, woman at 34-weeks' gestation comes in for a prenatal check-up. She had an appointment last week which was canceled due to a family emergency. She appears tired but states that she is otherwise fine. She denies vaginal bleeding, contractions, or fluid leakage. She is still able to feel her baby kick throughout the day. Her only medications right now are folate supplements and metformin. She cut down her cigarette use but recently began smoking a pack a day since the family emergency. She denies alcohol use or other substances. Vitals are 110/70 mmHg, 90 bpm, 98.6 °F, 20 RR. Physical exam is within normal limits for her gestational age. On exam, fetal heart sounds are appreciable on Doppler. What is the next best step in management?

Answer: D. Biophysical profile

Explanation: The key to this question is to see that the patient is 34 weeks pregnant and has a risk factor for fetal abnormalities (diabetes). The next best step is antepartum fetal testing, such as a biophysical profile, which is the combination of a non–stress test and an ultrasound. The ultrasound can detect fetal breathing movements, fetal limb movements, fetal limb tone, and amniotic fluid volume. Each of the five components, if normal, will receive a score of 2; a total score of 8 to 10 is normal.

A. Quad screen → Incorrect. Screen done in the second trimester for aneuploidy disorders. 34 weeks' gestation is too late.

B. Amniocentesis → Incorrect. Amniocentesis is used to rule out genetic abnormalities or infection.

C. Pregnancy-associated plasma protein A and beta-hCG → Incorrect. This is a screening test done in the first trimester to rule out Down syndrome.

E. Fetal fibronectin test → Incorrect. The fetal fibronectin test is used to assess for risk of preterm delivery. If the test is positive, the patient is at risk of having a preterm delivery.

99 AR
Biophysical profile during pregnancy video

Obstetric Complications

*Hao-Hua Wu, Leo Wang, Rebecca W. Gao,
and Cynthia DeTata*

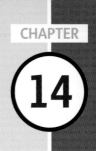
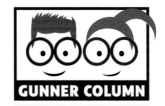

GUNNER COLUMN

Introduction

Obstetric complications are high-yield topics for the shelf. Although there is no official breakdown, expect to see at least 10 questions related to topics from this chapter on exam day. The four most frequently tested topics are spontaneous abortion, gestational diabetes, preeclampsia/eclampsia, and antepartum bleeding. Ectopic pregnancy and Rh incompatibility are also high-yield since they appear on the Medicine and Pediatric shelf exams as well.

This chapter is organized into (1) Spontaneous Abortion, (2) Medical Complications, (3) Antepartum Bleeding, and (4) Gunner Practice. Anticipate spending 8 to 12 hours to master the material and compare it with Chapter 8, which describes vaginal bleeding that occurs outside of pregnancy.

Spontaneous Abortion

Spontaneous abortion is defined as loss of a fetus at **less than 20 weeks' gestation**. Loss of a fetus at 20 weeks or later is known as a *stillbirth*. Vaginal bleeding is the chief complaint for spontaneous abortion, which consists of five types:

- *Complete abortion*: Passage of all products of conception, empty uterus on ultrasound (U/S), cervix open or closed
- *Incomplete abortion*: Passage of some products of conception, cervix open
- *Inevitable abortion*: No passage of products of conception but cervix open
- *Threatened abortion*: No passage of products of conception, cervix closed, but vaginal bleeding
- *Missed abortion*: No passage of products of conception, cervix closed, but intrauterine fetal death; possibly no bleeding

There are many risk factors for spontaneous abortion, but the high-yield ones for the shelf are those where prophylactic measures can be taken. These include:

QUICK TIP

Inevitable and incomplete = open os. Threatened and missed = closed os.

- Polycystic ovarian syndrome (PCOS) due to hyperglycemia → metformin
- Antiphospholipid syndrome → aspirin, heparin, low-molecular-weight heparin (LMWH)
- Asherman syndrome → lysis of adhesions
- Fibroids → myomectomy
- Cervical insufficiency → cerclage and vaginal progesterone
- Septate uterus → surgery (i.e., hysteroscopic metroplasty)
- Cigarette smoking → counseling to quit smoking

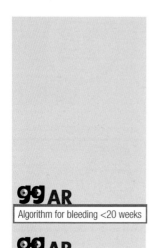

99 AR

Algorithm for bleeding <20 weeks

99 AR

APGO videos

Complete Abortion

Buzz Words: Occurs at <20 weeks gestation + passage of whole conceptus through the cervix + cervix then closes + associated pain and uterine contractions subside + U/S shows an empty uterus → complete abortion

Clinical Presentation: *Complete abortion* means that all the products of conception have been expelled from the uterus. This is the least commonly tested subgroup of spontaneous abortion since it is very easy to differentiate (it is the only subgroup where the uterus is empty on ultrasound). The urine beta-hCG will still be positive but the serum beta-hCG will gradually become undetectable by 4–6 weeks. The "solid white mass covered with blood" on the question stem represents the passage of embryonic or fetal tissue.

Prophylaxis (PPx): See introduction

Mechanism of Disease (MoD): Unknown but risk factors include maternal smoking, advanced maternal age, previous spontaneous abortion, and lethal structural/chromosomal abnormality of the fetus.

Diagnostic Steps (Dx):

1. Pelvic exam to check cervical os
2. Urine beta-hCG
3. Complete blood count (CBC) to determine degree of blood loss
4. Transvaginal ultrasound (TVUS)
5. Rh status

Treatment and Management Steps (Tx/Mgmt):

1. None; counseling

Incomplete Abortion

Buzz Words: Occurs at <20 weeks' gestation + vaginal bleeding w/ passage of large clots + uterine cramps + products of conception visualized in cervical os and on U/S + **open cervix**

Clinical Presentation: *Incomplete abortion* means that some of the products of conception remain in the uterus even though some have already passed. Passage with large clots is observed, the os is open, and some products of conception may be seen protruding through the os. Uterine evacuation of the remaining conceptus is done for treatment.

PPx: None

MoD: Unknown but risk factors include maternal smoking, advanced maternal age, previous spontaneous abortion, and lethal structural/chromosomal abnormality of the fetus.

Dx:

1. Same as for complete abortion:
   - Pelvic exam to check cervical os
   - Urine beta-hCG
   - CBC to determine degree of blood loss
   - TVUS
   - Rh status

Tx/Mgmt:

1. If hemoglobin levels are unstable → dilation and curettage (D + C), dilation and suction.
2. If hemoglobin levels are stable → prostaglandins (e.g., misoprostol), antiprogesterone (e.g., mifepristone).
3. If woman declines medical/surgical intervention and hemoglobin levels are stable → expectant management and close follow-up.

Inevitable Abortion

Buzz Words: Occurs at <20 weeks' gestation + vaginal bleeding + uterine cramps + possible intrauterine fetus with heartbeat still present + open cervical os

Clinical Presentation: *Inevitable abortion* is when all the products of conception are still in the uterus but the cervical os is open, indicating that an abortion is inevitable. Sometimes the question stem will state that the fetal heartbeat is still visible on ultrasound.

PPx: None

MoD: Unknown, but risk factors include maternal smoking, advanced maternal age, previous spontaneous abortion, and lethal structural/chromosomal abnormality of the fetus.

Dx:

1. Same as for complete abortion

Tx/Mgmt:

1. If hemoglobin levels are unstable → D + C, dilatation and suction.

2. If hemoglobin levels are stable and fetal age is <12 weeks → prostaglandins (e.g., misoprostol), antiprogesterone (e.g., mifepristone).
3. If woman declines medical/surgical intervention and hemoglobin levels are stable → expectant management and close follow-up.

Threatened Abortion

Buzz Words: Occurs at <20 weeks gestation + vaginal bleeding + fetal heartbeat present + closed cervical os

Clinical Presentation: In *threatened abortion*, there is no passage of products of conception and the cervical os is closed; however, vaginal bleeding suggests the risk of abortion. Threatened abortion can progress to inevitable, incomplete, and missed abortion.

PPx: Progesterone to prevent spontaneous abortion in women with recurrent spontaneous abortions (e.g., history of three or more)

MoD: Unknown, but risk factors include maternal smoking, advanced maternal age, previous spontaneous abortion, and lethal structural/chromosomal abnormality of the fetus.

Dx:
1. Same as for complete abortion

Tx/Mgmt:
1. Pelvic ultrasound to make sure fetus is alive and present → f/u with U/S again 1 week later.
2. Counseling and expectant management until resolution of symptoms or progression to inevitable, incomplete, or missed spontaneous abortion.

Missed Abortion

Buzz Words: Occurs at <20 weeks gestation + no vaginal bleeding + no fetal heartbeat present + closed cervical os

Clinical Presentation: *Missed abortion* is a pregnancy with no fetal heart tones and no symptoms of pregnancy loss (no bleeding, no pain, no open os—most often picked up on routine ultrasound or fetal heart tone check at ob appointment). Easy to pick out on the question stem because it is the only subgroup of abortion with no bleeding and a nonviable pregnancy demonstrated on U/S. Treatment algorithm is similar to inevitable and incomplete abortion.

PPx: None

MoD: Unknown but risk factors include maternal smoking, advanced maternal age, previous spontaneous abortion, and lethal structural/chromosomal abnormality of the fetus

Dx:
1. Same as for complete abortion
Tx/Mgmt:
1. If >12 weeks → D + C, dilation and suction
2. If <12 weeks → prostaglandins (e.g., misoprostol), anti-progesterone (e.g., mifepristone)
3. If woman declines medical/surgical intervention → expectant management

Stillbirth

Buzz Words: Occurs at ≥20 weeks gestation + nonviable pregnancy (intrauterine fetal demise [IUFD])
Clinical Presentation: *Stillbirth* refers to fetal death >20 weeks, in contrast to spontaneous abortion, which is fetal death <20 weeks. Be aware of this terminology in case you run into a question stem that shows nonviable pregnancy after a 20-week gestation.
PPx: Same as for spontaneous abortion
MoD: Many medical illnesses—such as diabetes, systemic lupus erythematosus (SLE), thyroid storm, severe maternal infection such as pneumonia or pyelonephritis, intrauterine infection, pregnancy-related disease such as preeclampsia, intrahepatic cholestasis of pregnancy (IHCP), or acute fatty liver of pregnancy (AFLP)—can lead to stillbirth. Lethal structural/chromosomal abnormality of the fetus can also lead to stillbirth.
Dx:
1. Same as for spontaneous abortion
Tx/Mgmt:
1. If second trimester:
   - 20–24 weeks → D + E or induction of labor depending on access to care
   - >24 weeks → induction of labor or spontaneous vaginal delivery
2. If third trimester → induction of labor and cervical ripening agents for spontaneous vaginal delivery; C-section if history of prior C-section.

Medical Complications

Acute Fatty Liver of Pregnancy

Buzz Words: Pregnant + fat droplets in hepatocytes (on autopsy) + acute liver function test (LFT) elevation in third trimester + N/V + abdominal pain + acute kidney injury (AKI)
Clinical Presentation: Fatty liver of pregnancy is an acute disorder that occurs close to term. The chief complaint is nausea and vomiting (N/V) and abdominal pain. Doctors may notice jaundice and see elevated LFTs on

AR

Intrahepatic cholestasis of pregnancy

lab. Outcomes range from self-limited to death of both patient and fetus. This topic is not commonly tested but may appear as an answer choice to rule out.

Dx:

1. CBC, basic metabolic panel (BMP), LFTs

Tx/Mgmt:

1. Immediate delivery and intensive treatment

Intrahepatic Cholestasis of Pregnancy

Buzz Words: Pregnant + **intense pruritus,** especially on the **palms and soles** + itching increased at night + elevated bilirubin + elevated LFTs + no visible rash

Clinical Presentation: The hallmark of intrahepatic cholestasis of pregnancy (ICP) is **pruritus** during pregnancy, which is seen in this disorder and not in AFLP. It occurs due to elevated bilirubin from hormone imbalance. Largely presents in the second and third trimesters and can be treated with Ursodeoxycholic acid.

MoD: Elevated bilirubin due to physiology of pregnancy

Dx:

1. CBC, BMP, and liver panel
2. Fasting total serum bile acid level

Tx/Mgmt:

1. Ursodeoxycholic acid

Anemia of Pregnancy

Buzz Words:

- **Dilutional anemia:** No other symptoms; out of proportion with stage of pregnancy
- **Iron-deficiency anemia:** Microcytic + low iron/ferritin
- **Alpha thalassemia:** Microcytic + normal iron + Asian mother + hydrops fetalis
- **B12 deficiency:** Macrocytic + peripheral neurologic symptoms
- Folate deficiency: Macrocytic

Clinical Presentation: The differential for anemia of pregnancy on the shelf can be divided into three categories: (1) dilutional anemia, (2) microcytic anemia, and (3) macrocytic anemia. No treatment or further evaluation is needed if the hemoglobin is between 10 and 12 g/dL. Further workup is required for patients with <10 hgb, which includes determination of mean cell volume (MCV) and folate/B12 levels if macrocytic (MCV >100) or Fe levels and electrophoresis for thalassemia if microcytic (MCV <100). Treatment depends on the disorder.

The most important take-home point is being able to distinguish normal from abnormal anemia of pregnancy.

PPx: N/A

MoD:

- Normal anemia of pregnancy can occur when the rate of plasma volume increases faster than the rate of RBC volume. (Patient remains asymptomatic and does not need intervention.)
- Fe-deficiency anemia due to inadequate dietary intake and increased need (higher RBC volume)
- Folate-deficiency anemia due to inadequate dietary intake and increased need (higher RBC volume)

Dx:

1. CBC with MCV
   - If MCV >100 → folate and B12 levels to r/o macrocytic anemia
   - If MCV<80 → iron labs to r/o Fe deficiency + electrophoresis to r/o hemoglobinopathies

Tx/Mgmt: Depends on etiology

1. Replete Fe, folate, or B12 as needed.
2. If the patient has sickle cell disease and is severely ill (e.g., heart failure, septic shock), perform exchange transfusions. Avoid hypoxemia (from asthma or respiratory infections—give flu vaccine) and hypovolemia (dehydration from nausea or diarrhea—give IV rehydration rapidly) to prevent sickling and painful episodes. Sickle cell crises can cause fetal growth problems, preterm labor, and intrauterine fetal demise. The father of the fetus should also be tested to determine whether the fetus has a hemoglobinopathy incompatible with life so that the family may consider the option of early termination.

Cardiac Conditions Worsened by Pregnancy

Buzz Words:

- **Mitral stenosis:** Opening snap with late diastolic rumble
- **Aortic stenosis:** Harsh crescendo-decrescendo mid-systolic murmur
- **Heart failure:** Elevated jugular venous pressure + lower extremity edema + crackles on lung exam + orthopnea

Clinical Presentation: In normal pregnancy, cardiac output is increased (e.g., increased HR and stroke volume) to accommodate for the placenta and fetus. Increased stroke volume and HR can exacerbate existing cardiac conditions such as heart failure, mitral stenosis, and aortic stenosis. Some patients with preexisting cardiac pathology may begin to show signs on exam (e.g., harsh midsystolic murmur for aortic stenosis) that you will likely be asked to identify.

PPx: Some cardiac conditions can worsen markedly with pregnancy. Patients should understand risk before conceiving, should be offered appropriate and effective contraception, and should be offered termination if they become pregnant by accident or without knowing the risks. Patients should undergo treatment for any heart condition prior to pregnancy.

MoD: Physiologically, pregnant women have higher heart rates and stroke volumes, leading to greater cardiac output and more strain on the heart, thereby exacerbating conditions like mitral/aortic stenosis. In some conditions, the most dangerous part of pregnancy is immediately after delivery with the autoshunting of blood from the uterus.

Dx:
1. Electrocardiogram (ECG)
2. Echocardiogram (Echo)

Tx/Mgmt:
1. Optimize diuretics, timing of delivery, ICU care for heart failure patients.

Cervical Insufficiency (aka Cervical Incompetence)

Buzz Words: >20 weeks + open, soft cervix or shortened cervix (<2.5 cm) + preterm delivery

Clinical Presentation: Cervical insufficiency is a disorder of the cervix where the musculature is not strong enough to keep the cervix closed until term. Patients with cervical insufficiency are at risk for preterm labor and delivery (20–37 weeks' gestation). The classic presentation is a patient with preterm delivery found to have an open, soft cervix <2.5 cm on exam or ultrasound. Be sure to differentiate this from the types of spontaneous abortions (e.g., incomplete and inevitable), which occur <20 weeks gestation. Cervical insufficiency is idiopathic and is associated with bicornuate/septate uterus, excessive dilation with previous surgical intervention, prior cone biopsies, and diseases of collagen synthesis (e.g., Marfan syndrome).

PPx: Weekly TVUS after 16 weeks if patient has risk factors for cervical insufficiency. Prophylactic cerclage midway through pregnancy if patient has a history of cervical insufficiency.

MoD: Unknown; weakness of cervical tissue

Dx:
1. Clinical presentation (no contractions but may have pinkish discharge, open os)
2. Pelvic ultrasound
3. Transvaginal ultrasound

99 AR

Cervical insufficiency

Tx/Mgmt:
1. Cerclage
2. Vaginal progesterone

Ectopic Pregnancy

Buzz Words:
- **Ectopic pregnancy:** Abdominal pain + amenorrhea + vaginal bleeding + palpable adnexal mass
- **Ectopic pregnancy:** Beta-hCG >2000 + nothing in the uterus + no fetal pole in uterus
- **Ruptured ectopic pregnancy:** Abdominal pain + amenorrhea + vaginal bleeding + orthostatic changes + hypovolemic shock

99 AR
Ectopic pregnancy

Clinical Presentation: Ectopic pregnancy is a condition in which the fertilized egg matures outside of the uterus (e.g., in the fallopian tube). This can present as abdominal pain and be mistaken for a GI disorder. Patient with hypotension and tachycardia suggests a ruptured ectopic pregnancy and requires immediate admission and surgery. Risk factors include previous ectopic/pelvic/tubal surgery, infertility treatments, use of an intrauterine device (IUD), pelvic inflammatory disease (PID), and multiple sexual partners.

MoD: Ectopic pregnancy is caused by failure of a fertilized egg to implant in the endometrium. Most often occurs in the ampulla of the fallopian tube.

Dx:
1. Pelvic exam
2. Quantitative (NOT qualitative) beta-hCG
3. Pelvic ultrasound (no fetus or sac visualized in uterus)

Tx/Mgmt:
1. If hemodynamically stable, methotrexate. Trend beta-hCG every 2 days with close follow-up.
2. If unstable, emergent surgery.

Gestational Diabetes

Buzz Words:
- **Maternal complications** = gestational diabetes + polyhydramnios + preeclampsia + spontaneous abortion + difficult labor
- **Fetal complications** = shoulder dystocia + hypocalcemia + hypoglycemia + polycythemia + neural tube defects + hyperbilirubinemia + enlarged organs + growth abnormalities + intrauterine fetal demise

99 AR
Gestational diabetes management

Clinical Presentation: Gestational diabetes causes elevated blood glucose levels during pregnancy. It is thought to be due to insulin resistance arising from hPL, estrogen, and progesterone. For prenatal care, it is routine to screen for gestational diabetes with an HgbA1c and oral glucose tolerance test. Control of blood sugar is important to minimize maternal complications (e.g., polyhydramnios + spontaneous abortion + preeclampsia) and fetal complications (e.g., macrosomia + hypoglycemia + polycythemia + neural tube defects) that may occur. On the shelf, make sure to know the complications well (included in the buzz words).

An important concept to consider is that maternal hyperglycemia can affect the fetus differently depending on the trimester. If the mother has gestational diabetes during the **first trimester**, she is at risk for spontaneous abortion, while the fetus is at risk for small left colon syndrome (inability to pass meconium), neural tube defects, and congenital heart disease.

If the mother has gestational diabetes during the **second and third trimester**, the fetus develops **hyperinsulinemia,** leading to four main complications:

- Macrosomia (big body), which can lead to traumatic birth injuries like shoulder dystocia, Erb palsy, and brachial plexus injury
- Big organs (e.g., cardiomegaly)
- Polycythemia due to more RBC mass to supply the enlarged organs, jaundice, hyperbilirubinemia, kernicterus as the RBCs break down
- **Hypo**glycemia as a neonate

PPx:

- Oral glucose tolerance test (OGTT): 50 g load + measurement at 1 hour → if blood glucose >130 mg/dL, give a second test with a 100 g load and measure at 3 hours
- Nonstress tests, biophysical profiles, and kick counts after 32 weeks
- Postpartum screening and insulin levels

MoD: Unknown but associated with insulin resistance that can arise from the influence of human placental lactogen (hPL), estrogen, and progesterone

Dx:

1. OGTT
2. Plasma glucose (two fasting readings >126 mg/dL)
3. Hemoglobin A1c for existing diabetics

Tx/Mgmt:

1. Blood glucose daily monitoring
2. Insulin
3. Glyburide
4. If PCOS, give metformin
5. Induce if >39 weeks
6. C-section if severe macrosomia

QUICK TIP

Newborns of patients with gestational diabetes have **hypo**glycemia because of the **hyper**insulinemia compensating for the mother's high blood sugar. Once the newborn is no longer attached by the umbilical cord, the ratio of insulin to blood sugar becomes too high.

Polyhydramnios

Buzz Words: Amniotic fluid index >25 cm + preterm labor + uterine atony + maternal (gestational) diabetes

Clinical Presentation: Polyhydramnios is a condition where there is excessive amniotic fluid as measured by U/S. The excess fluid can be indicative of impaired swallowing mechanism (e.g., tracheoesophageal fistula, other GI abnormalities). In normal gestation, the fetus is able to swallow the fluid, which is recirculated through the placental and maternal circulation. Without the swallowing mechanism, the fluid accumulates and can lead to preterm labor as well as uterine atony because of overstretching of the uterus, leading the body to think that the gestational age is greater than it is.

MoD: Defective GI tract → fetus cannot swallow amniotic fluid → buildup of amniotic fluid

Dx:

1. U/S to observe amniotic fluid index (>25 cm) and fetal malformation

Tx/Mgmt:

1. Mild to moderate:
   - Nonstress test and biophysical profile every 1–2 weeks until 37 weeks
   - Induction of labor at 37 weeks
2. Severe:
   - Indomethacin if <32 weeks
   - Amnioreduction if 32–34 weeks
   - Induction of labor if >34 weeks

> **QUICK TIP**
>
> Gestational diabetes can cause polyhydramnios due to increased fluid production.

Oligohydramnios

Buzz Words: Amniotic fluid index <5 cm + **pulmonary hypoplasia** + **postterm** pregnancy

Clinical Presentation: Oligohydramnios is a condition of reduced levels of amniotic fluid associated with postterm births. For the fetus, it is associated with fetal demise, pulmonary hypoplasia (since amniotic fluid is needed for lung development), limb contractures, and growth restrictions.

MoD:

- **Second trimester:** Kidney makes amniotic fluid; kidney defects or obstruction. Examples of causes of fetal kidney problems include hypoxia (less O_2 → shunting blood away from kidney).
- **Third trimester:** Preterm premature rupture of membranes, uteroplacental insufficiency, fetal anomalies.

Dx:

1. Ultrasound to observe amniotic fluid index (>25 cm) and fetal malformation

2. Nitrazine test to r/o rupture of membranes
3. Doppler of umbilical artery if suspected uteroplacental insufficiency
4. amniocentesis for karyotyping

Tx/Mgmt:
1. Counseling
2. Serial ultrasound (1 per 4 weeks)
3. Induction of labor at 37 weeks

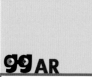
Kleihauer-Betke test video

Hypertension During Pregnancy

Chronic hypertension, gestational hypertension, preeclampsia, eclampsia, and chronic hypertension with preeclampsia are on the differential anytime there is a BP >140/>90 on the shelf. The way to think of these disorders is on a continuum:

- **Chronic hypertension (HTN)** is >140/>90 mm Hg at **<20 weeks'** gestation or before pregnancy.
- **Gestational hypertension** is new-onset >140/>90 mm Hg at **>20 weeks** gestation + no end-organ damage or proteinuria.
- **Preeclampsia** is new-onset >140/>90 mm Hg at **>20 weeks** gestation + end-organ damage or proteinuria.
- **Chronic HTN with preeclampsia** is chronic HTN with signs of end-organ damage, worsening proteinuria >20 weeks, or acute exacerbation of HTN.
- **Eclampsia** is preeclampsia + new onset seizures (grand mal).

Treatment of HTN can be done by methyldopa, labetalol, nifedipine, thiazide, or clonidine. Avoid antihypertensives that damage the kidneys (e.g., angiotensin-converting enzyme [ACE] inhibitors, angiotensin receptor blockers [ARBs], aldosterone blockers, furosemide, renin blockers).

Gestational Hypertension

Buzz Words: New HTN (140/90) in pregnant women >20 weeks + NO proteinuria + otherwise normal

Tx/Mgmt:
1. Antihypertensives and close follow-up

Mild Preeclampsia

Buzz Words: New HTN (140/90) in pregnant woman >20 weeks + proteinuria

Clinical Presentation: A gravida 1 para 0 female at 30 weeks' gestation presents to prenatal clinic with two BP readings of 150/90 and 500 mg protein on 24-hour urine collection. Creatinine is normal and she has no other laboratory or physical exam abnormalities.

Preeclampsia and Eclampsia. APGO.

PPx: Risk factors include past history of preeclampsia (personal or familial), first pregnancy, obesity, CKD, diabetes, advanced maternal age, multiple gestations.

Dx:
1. Urine analysis:
   a. Dipstick (protein)
   b. 24-hour urine collection (>300 mg protein, protein/Cr >0.3)
2. BMP (normal Cr)
3. CBC (normal)
4. LFTs (normal)

Tx/Mgmt:
1. Antihypertensives and close follow-up
2. Induce labor at 37 weeks (C-section is not necessary.)

Preeclampsia With Severe Features

Buzz Words: BP 160/110 + swelling of face/hands + proteinuria + thrombocytopenia <100k + pulmonary edema + signs of end-organ damage (headache, visual changes, epigastric pain, altered mental status, dyspnea)

Clinical Presentation: A gravida 1 para 0 female at 30 weeks' gestation presents to her prenatal clinic visit with a BP of 170/120, a creatinine of 1.5, thrombocytopenia, cough, headache, and abdominal pain.

PPx: Same risk factors as preeclampsia without severe features

Dx:
1. Urine analysis:
   a. Dipstick (protein)
   b. 24-hour urine collection (>5000 mg protein)
2. BMP (Cr >1.1)
3. CBC (thrombocytopenia)
4. LFTs (elevated)
5. CXR (pulmonary edema)

Tx/Mgmt:
1. Magnesium sulfate for seizure prophylaxis
2. Antihypertensive medications (to prevent stroke)
3. Induce labor at 34 weeks (C-section is not necessary.)

Superimposed Preeclampsia

Buzz Words: Preeclampsia in a woman with chronic HTN even before pregnancy

Eclampsia

Buzz Words: Seizures in pregnant woman

Clinical Presentation: Seizures in a pregnant woman >20 weeks' gestation

QUICK TIP
On the Ob/Gyn shelf, there is only one disorder (eclampsia) that presents as seizures while pregnant.

PPx: Same risk factors as preeclampsia but without severe features

Dx:
1. Clinical diagnosis based on presence of seizures

Tx/Mgmt:
1. Stabilize mother (intubate if respiratory collapse)
2. IV magnesium sulfate
3. Emergency C-section

HELLP Syndrome

Definition: Hemolysis, Elevated LFTs, and Low Platelet count (HELLP syndrome)

Buzz Words: Schistocytes + elevated bilirubin + low haptoglobin + elevated LDH + elevated LFTs (AST or ALT 2x upper limit of normal) + <100K platelets + epigastric pain and vomiting

Clinical Presentation: Note that HTN is not mandatory for the diagnosis of HELLP.

PPx: Risk factors include previous personal history of HELLP or preeclampsia.

Dx:
1. CBC (<100K platelets)
2. Peripheral smear (schistocytes)
3. LFT (AST and ALT 2x upper limit of normal, elevated bilirubin)

Tx/Mgmt:
1. Magnesium sulfate
2. Immediate delivery if >34 weeks. Delivery after corticosteroids if <34 weeks.
3. Supportive care (ABCs, transfuse platelets, manage HTN, etc.)

Hyperemesis Gravidarum

Buzz Words: Losing weight during pregnancy + nausea/vomiting + weakness/lightheadedness + dry mucous membranes + orthostatic vital signs (volume-depleted) + cannot tolerate PO at all

Clinical Presentation: Hyperemesis gravidarum is a disorder where the patient experiences intractable nausea and vomiting during pregnancy.

Dx:
1. BMP, CBC
2. Orthostatic vital signs
3. Thyroid functioning tests
4. UA
5. Pelvic ultrasound to r/o hydatidiform mole and multiple gestations

QUICK TIP

RUQ/epigastric pain due to **distension of the liver capsule** aka (Glisson's capsule); schistocytes due to microangiopathic hemolytic anemia

99 AR

HELLP syndrome

Tx/Mgmt:
1. Admission for IV hydration and antiemetic therapy
2. Pyridoxine
3. Antiemetics (e.g., chlorpromazine)

Rh Isoimmunization for Incompatibility

Buzz Words:
- Rh- mother + Rh+ fetus
- **Erythroblastosis fetalis:** Mother's second pregnancy + neonatal unconjugated hyperbilirubinemia + neonatal anemia + neonatal positive Coombs test

Clinical Presentation: *Rh incompatibility* refers to the phenomenon whereby an Rh- mother develops antibodies to Rh factor from carrying an Rh+ fetus. Although this mismatch **does not affect the first pregnancy,** the second pregnancy with an Rh+ fetus is at risk for erythroblastosis fetalis, or hemolytic anemia of the fetus due to attack from maternal RBC antibodies. Prophylactic measures, known as Rh isoimmunization, will likely be represented by one or two questions on the shelf. Make sure to know the indications for anti-D immunoglobulin administration to an unsensitized Rh- mother, which would include the following:
1. First dose at 28-weeks' gestation
2. Second dose within 72 hours of delivering Rh+ infant (e.g., live birth, stillborn, spontaneous abortion)
3. Ectopic pregnancy
4. Vaginal bleeding in the second and third trimesters
5. Amniocentesis
6. Trauma

PPx: If woman is Rh-, anti-D immunoglobulin administration at 28 weeks pregnancy and within 72 hours of delivery, stillborn or spontaneous abortion

MoD: Rh- mother and Rh+ father make Rh+ fetus → mother's immune system develops antibodies to Rh factor → Rh+ antibodies attack fetal red blood cells → erythroblastosis fetalis

Dx:
1. RhD antigen test for fetus and mother to determine Rh status.
2. Kleihauer–Betke test to determine how much anti-D immunoglobulin will be needed postpartum.

Tx/Mgmt:
1. C-section

FOR THE WARDS
Anti-D immunoglobulin is called RhoGAM on the wards.

FOR THE WARDS
Anti-D given at Twen-D-eight weeks

FOR THE WARDS
Erythroblastosis fetalis = hemolytic anemia of the neonate due to maternal RBC antibodies

Antepartum Hemorrhage, Including Third-Trimester Bleeding

Vaginal bleeding during the third trimester requires workup to r/o potentially life-threatening pathology. The four most important etiologies of third-trimester bleeding are (1) abruptio placentae, (2) vasa previa, (3) placenta previa, and (4) rupture of the uterus. Be able to use buzz words to distinguish these four entities on the shelf. Last, remember that one can expect to see a "bloody show" during normal pregnancy, which heralds the onset of labor.

Abruptio Placentae (Placental Abruption)

Buzz Words:
- HTN/cocaine/meth use+ **painful bleeding in the third trimester** + contractions + hypertonic uterus + abdominal pain
- Abdominal trauma (e.g., car accident) + abdominal pain

Clinical Presentation: Placental abruption is a disorder defined by premature separation of placenta from uterus and is often considered to be an emergency. The classic presentation on the shelf is a third-trimester patient who presents with **painful vaginal bleeding.** Sometimes you will be shown an accompanying fetal heart tracing showing fetal distress (e.g., tachycardia, late decelerations, no improvement with intrauterine resuscitation measures).

The trickiest aspect of this disorder is that the patient may not always present with vaginal bleeding! Bleeding from the rupture may be concealed because the hemorrhage is contained behind the placenta. Any abdominal trauma or sudden abdominal pain in a third-trimester patient should raise red flags.

PPx: Treatment of HTN. Tobacco cessation.

MoD: Associated with many factors, including factor V Leiden, hypertension, multiparity, prolonged premature rupture of membranes, tobacco use, trauma, and cocaine. From this list only memorize the ones that can be prevented for the shelf, as you may be tested on prophylactic management.

Dx:
1. Pelvic exam and pelvic ultrasound
2. Fetal heart rate (FHR) monitoring
3. Apt test (to differentiate fetal from maternal blood)

Tx/Mgmt:
1. Rh immunoglobulins if patient is Rh-negative.
2. IV fluids.

---

99 AR
Algorithm for third trimester bleeding.

99 AR
Normal and abdominal bleeding. APGO.

99 AR
Third-trimester bleeding. APGO.

QUICK TIP
Differential for third trimester bleeding: Painless = vasa previa, placenta previa. Painful = placental rupture.

QUICK TIP
Sudden loss of fetal station = placental rupture on the shelf

QUICK TIP
Apt test shows pink fluid after hemolysis → fetal blood; Apt test shows yellow-brown fluid after hemolysis → maternal blood

3. RBCs and plasma transfer.
4. If mother and fetus are both stable + cervix fully dilated → vaginal delivery.
5. If mother and fetus are unstable + cervix not fully dilated → emergent C-section.

Vasa Previa

Buzz Words: **Painless** vaginal bleeding right after rupture of membranes (both natural and artificial) + fetal distress on monitor + fetal sinusoidal pattern (for severe anemia) + normal maternal vital signs

Clinical Presentation: Vasa previa is a disorder characterized by fetal blood vessels that overlie the cervical os and are at risk for rupture if baby is delivered. Vasa previa is **emergent** because rupture of these vessels, which connect cord to placenta, could lead to fetal demise due to hemorrhage. Chief complaint is usually **painless light-red vaginal bleeding** in the third trimester s/p rupture of membranes. But don't let the "painless" bleeding lull you into complacency; on the shelf, emergent C-section is the preferred first-line treatment.

PPx: Delivery at 35 weeks by planned C-section to avoid the risk of rupture even if no bleeding has occurred.

Dx:
1. Pelvic exam and pelvic ultrasound
2. FHR monitoring
3. Apt test (to differentiate fetal from maternal blood)

Tx/Mgmt:
1. Emergent C-section

Placenta Previa

Buzz Words: **Painless** vaginal bleeding in **third trimester** s/p digital vaginal exam or sex + low-lying placenta

Clinical Presentation: *Placenta previa* refers to abnormal implantation of the placenta either directly over the internal cervical os or near enough to obstruct the opening. Like vasa previa, it may present with painless vaginal bleeding in the third trimester. If patient does have massive hemorrhage after diagnosis of placenta previa, bleeding can be associated with concomitant placental abruption or disseminated intravascular coagulopathy (DIC).

MoD: Associated with prior C-section, multiparity, advanced age, and multiple gestation

Dx:
1. Ultrasound (abdominal then vaginal)
2. FHR monitoring

Uterine rupture

Note: Digital exams are CONTRAINDICATED due to risk of causing hemorrhage.

Tx/Mgmt:
1. If hemodynamically stable mother and fetus → elective C-section
2. If unstable mother and fetus → emergent C-section
3. If <34 weeks, steroids to promote fetal lung maturity

Uterine Rupture

Buzz Words: Prior C-section + **third trimester** + sudden intense lower abdominal pain + **fetal head shifts from lower to higher station** (e.g., +1 to −1) + protuberance felt in belly + repetitive variable decelerations + bradycardia

Clinical Presentation: Rupture of the uterus during labor can occur, leading to massive hemorrhage. This is often associated with prior insult to the uterus, including traumatic injury (e.g., car crash) or scarring due to previous surgery or infection. This is a life-threatening emergency and should be managed by immediate C-section. A classic presentation is a mother pushing in active labor when suddenly the fetal head goes from +1 to −2 station.

MoD: Associated with prior C-sections, multiparity, advanced age, and multiple gestations

Dx:
1. Ultrasound (abdominal, then vaginal)
2. FHR monitoring

Tx/Mgmt:
1. C-section
2. If <34 weeks, steroids to promote fetal lung maturity

GUNNER PRACTICE

1. A 24-year-old, gravida 1, para 0, woman at 19 weeks' gestation comes to her physician complaining of vaginal bleeding for the last 2 days. No pain. She denies any recent trauma although does admit to having had sexual intercourse with her husband 2 weeks earlier. Her medications include iron supplements and a daily multivitamin. She does not smoke or drink and continues to work as a sales representative. Her vitals are 120/80 mm Hg, 95 bpm, 99 °F, and 14 RR. On exam, there is scant blood in the vaginal canal, and her cervix is closed. She does not have any tenderness to palpation of her uterus or adnexa. A complete blood count shows no abnormalities and a fetal heart rate is heard on Doppler. What is the most likely diagnosis?
A. Placental abruption
B. Vasa previa

C. Threatened abortion

D. Inevitable abortion

E. Missed abortion

2. A 32-year-old, gravida 3, para 2, woman at 31 weeks' gestation presents to her physician with facial edema and headache. Her prenatal course is complicated by high readings on the oral glucose tolerance test, for which she is now taking insulin. This is also her first pregnancy with an Rh+ fetus, and she was given anti-D immunoglobulin 3 weeks ago. A former heavy drinker, she still has about a beer a week. She continues her work as a substitute teacher, although she sometimes still experiences intense bouts of nausea in the middle of class. Her vitals are 150/100 mm Hg, 95 bpm, 99 °F, 14 RR, and 99% on room air. During the exam, her extremities turn stiff and she begins to convulse. She is taken to the emergency department for stabilization. What is the most appropriate next step in management?

A. Valproic acid

B. Ethosuximide

C. Basic metabolic panel

D. Corticosteroids

E. Magnesium

3. A 29-year-old, gravida 2, para 1, female at 36 weeks' gestation comes to the physician complaining of several episodes of painless postcoital vaginal bleeding, which has resolved. Her only medications are iron supplements and a multivitamin pill. Her last pregnancy was complicated by gestational diabetes, which resolved a few weeks after delivery. Her vitals are 120/60 mm Hg, 90 HR, 99°F, 18 RR, and 96% on room air. What is the most appropriate management?

A. C-section at term

B. Emergent C-section

C. Vaginal delivery at term

D. Induction of labor

E. Misoprostol

ANSWER: What Would Gunner Jess/Jim Do?

1. **WWGJD?** A 24-year-old, gravida 1, para 0, woman at **19 weeks' gestation** comes to her physician complaining of **vaginal bleeding** for the last 2 days. No pain. She denies any recent trauma although does admit to having sexual intercourse with her husband 2 weeks ago. Her medications include iron supplements and a daily multivitamin. She does not smoke or drink, and continues to work as a sales representative. Her vitals are 120/80, 95 bpm, 99°F, and 14 RR. On exam, there is scant blood in the vaginal canal, and her **cervix is closed.** She does not have any tenderness to palpation of her uterus or adnexa. A complete blood count shows no abnormalities. **Fetal heart beat is heard faintly on Doppler. What is the most likely diagnosis?**

Answer: C. Threatened abortion

Explanation: Because this is vaginal bleeding occurring **before 20 weeks' gestation**, suspect some type of spontaneous abortion. Right away, you can rule out placental abruption and vasa previa, which tend to occur during the third trimester. Thus you are left with the subgroups of spontaneous abortion. Remember, the first step is to check whether the os is open or closed. Closed os eliminates inevitable abortion. To distinguish between threatened and missed, look for the presence of vaginal bleeding as well as fetal heart activity. Missed abortion can be ruled out because there is both vaginal bleeding and fetal heart activity. Thus threatened abortion is the answer. Ultrasound would have shown an entire conceptus in the uterus.

A. Placental abruption → Incorrect. Placental abruption presents with painful vaginal bleeding and late decelerations on fetal heart monitoring. It occurs after 20 weeks' gestation, so can be ruled out immediately.

B. Vasa previa → Incorrect. Vasa previa is vaginal bleeding due to rupture of fetal blood vessels that overlie cervical os. This occurs after 20 weeks' gestation and can be ruled out immediately.

D. Inevitable abortion → Incorrect. Inevitable abortion presents with an open cervix and presence of the entire conceptus within the uterus. It can be ruled out as soon as you see "cervix closed" on the questions stem.

E. Missed abortion → Incorrect. Missed abortion has vaginal bleeding but **not in the presence of**

the clinician. Also, the pregnancy is always non-viable. Thus this is incorrect, as fetal heartbeats were heard.

2. WWGJD? A 32-year-old, gravida 3, para 2, woman at 31 weeks' gestation presents to her physician with facial edema and headache. Her prenatal course is complicated by high readings on the oral glucose tolerance test, for which she is now taking insulin. This is also her first pregnancy with an Rh+ fetus, and she was given anti-D immunoglobulin 3 weeks ago. A former heavy drinker, she still has about one beer a week. She continues her work as a substitute teacher, although she sometimes still experiences intense bouts of nausea in the middle of class. Her vitals are 150/100 mm Hg, 95 bpm, 99°F, 14 RR, and 99% on room air. During the exam, her extremities turn stiff and she begins to convulse. Patient is taken to the emergency department for stabilization. What is the most appropriate next step in management?

Answer: E. Magnesium

Explanation: It is likely that this patient is experiencing eclampsia, which occurs in patients with high blood pressure and either proteinuria or one sign of end-organ dysfunction (e.g., preeclampsia). The hallmark of eclampsia is a seizure during pregnancy, a buzz word not shared by any other entity on the Ob/Gyn shelf. First-line treatment for stabilization of these patients is intravenous magnesium.

A. Valproic acid → Incorrect. Although valproic acid is used for generalized tonic seizures, like the one the patient is experiencing, it is not used in pregnant patients due to the risk of teratogenicity.

B. Ethosuximide → Incorrect. Ethosuximide is an antiepileptic drug used to treat absence seizures (e.g., seizures where patients stop what they are doing for a few seconds and have no recollection of the event). It is not used for management of seizures from eclampsia.

C. Basic metabolic panel → Incorrect. A BMP would be a reasonable next step had this patient not seized, since it could help to confirm a diagnosis of preeclampsia (e.g., if Cr >1.1). However, seizures require prompt treatment.

D. Corticosteroids → Incorrect. Steroids are given to mothers whose fetuses are less than 34 weeks old to support lung maturation. Although patient may need this in the next few days if the fetus is being delivered prematurely, it is not the correct next step.

3. WWGJD? A 29-year-old, gravida 2, para 1, female at 36 weeks' gestation comes to the physician complaining of several episodes of painless postcoital vaginal bleeding, which resolved. Her only medications are iron supplements and a multivitamin pill. Her last pregnancy was complicated by gestational diabetes, which resolved a few weeks after delivery. Her vitals are 120/60 mm Hg, 90 HR, 99°F, 18 RR, and 96% on room air. What is the most appropriate management?

Answer: A. Elective C-section

Explanation: The key to this question is to recognize that the patient is in the third trimester with painless vaginal bleeding, suggestive of a placenta previa.

B. Emergency C-section → Incorrect. This patient is hemodynamically stable.

C. Vaginal delivery at term → Incorrect. This patient likely has a placenta previa, which would pose a very high risk of dangerous hemorrhage in a vaginal delivery.

D. Induction of labor → Incorrect. Same as above.

E. Misoprostol → Incorrect. Misoprostol is a prostaglandin analog used for the medical treatment of spontaneous abortion.

Labor and Delivery

Leo Wang and Hao-Hua Wu

Introduction

Although this chapter is very high-yield for your Ob/Gyn rotation, it is not high-yield for the shelf. As a clerkship student, you will be expected to know how to examine a woman in labor, determine cervical dilation, and know fancy maneuvers to facilitate delivery of the baby such as the Leopold maneuver. However, the normal process of delivering a baby will not be tested on the Ob/Gyn shelf (e.g., the topics covered in "Assessment of the Woman in Labor" and "The Labor Process"). Instead, question writers are more interested in how to identify when things are abnormal. The most commonly tested topic, for instance, is **how to tell whether there is a premature rupture of membranes: nitrazine paper turns blue from exposure to fluid.**

This chapter is organized into (1) Assessment of the Woman in Labor, (2) The Labor Process, (3) Complicated Labor and Delivery, and (4) Gunner Practice. Make sure to plan your studying wisely. If you know the normal process of delivery well, skip to the "Complicated Labor and Delivery" subsection. If you are just starting on your Ob/Gyn rotation and need background in order to look like an all-star on the L&D floor, peruse the first two subsections as well. Anticipate spending no more than 4–6 hours studying this material.

Assessment of the Woman in Labor

As mentioned in the intro, this section is not directly tested on the shelf, but knowing what's normal can help you understand the abnormal.

First, painful uterine contractions typically indicate labor, but other more obvious signs include membrane rupture in the form of bloody vaginal discharge or mucous plugging. Cervical dilation greater than 4 cm usually indicates labor. Upon admission to the floor, the first and most important step is to get an accurate pregnancy and obstetric history while also validating the medical and social history. Your initial workup should include vitals, weight, BMI, frequency

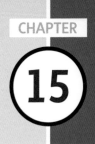

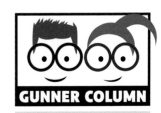

GUNNER COLUMN

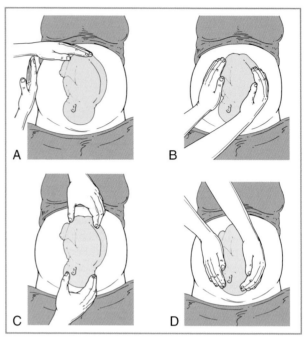

FIG. 15.1 The Leopold maneuver: antepartum fetal assessment and therapy. (A) First maneuver: Determine presenting part. (B) Second maneuver: Find fetal vertebrae. (C) Third maneuver: Determine fetal mobility. (D) Fourth maneuver: Determine fetal descent.

of contractions, quality, duration, and fetal heart rate. In addition, the most important part of your physical exam is the **obstetric examination**.

Your first goal in the obstetric examination is to determine fetal lie, fetal presentation, and conduct a cervical exam. **Fetal lie** tells you whether the infant is in a longitudinal or transverse position in the uterus. The **Leopold maneuver** is used to determine fetal lie (Fig. 15.1).

The Leopold maneuver consists of palpating first at the fundus, then on either side of the uterus, and then above the pubic symphysis to determine fetal lie. Fetal presentation should also be determined, specifically if the infant is in the breech or vertex position. This can be determined from palpation or from ultrasound (Fig. 15.2).

The cervical exam is the last component of the physical exam to be performed. First, determine if rupture of membranes has occurred. This is usually diagnosed from a history of leaking fluid from vagina and can be diagnosed from the nitrazine and fern tests. Nitrazine tests for alkaline amniotic fluid from vaginal secretions (amniotic fluid is more basic than vaginal secretions and turns the paper **blue**). The fern test looks for ferning of amniotic fluid under low microscopic power (Fig. 15.3).

Fetal Presentation

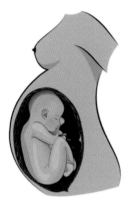 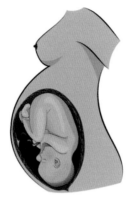

Breech Presentation   Vertex Presentation

FIG. 15.2 Fetal presentations.

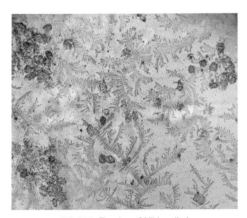

FIG. 15.3 Ferning. (Wikipedia.)

Rupture of the membranes occurs 1 hour before labor 10% of the time. If it occurs 18 hours before labor, this is considered premature rupture of membranes (PROM). If rupture of membranes occurs as early as 37 weeks, it is considered preterm, premature rupture of membranes (PPROM).

After determining if rupture of membranes has occurred, proceed with the remainder of the cervical exam by observing five characteristics that together make up what is known as the **Bishop Score**: position, consistency, effacement, dilation, and station (Table 15.1).

A bishop score of 8 or higher is good for spontaneous labor. Position refers to the cervical position. Consistency is self-explanatory. Effacement is how "thin" the cervix is and the thinner it is (>80%) the more prepared for delivery. Dilation is the size of the cervical os. Fetal station describes the position of the head relative to ischial spines. +1 and

TABLE 15.1 Bishop Score

Cervix	SCORE				Bishop Score Modifiers
	0	1	2	3	
Position	Posterior	Mid-posterior	Anterior		**Add 1 point for:**
Consistency	Firm	Medium	Soft		• Pre-eclampsia
Effacement	0%–30%	30%–50%	60%–70%	>80%	• Each previous vaginal delivery
Dilation	Closed	1–2 cm	3–4 cm	>5 cm	**Subtract 1 point for:**
Station	–3	–2	–1	+1, +2	• Postdate pregnancy
					• Nulliparity (no previous vaginal deliveries)
					• PPROM (preterm premature rupture of membranes)

Andrea Crossman, RN, holisticdoulanyc.com.

Stages of Labor

QUICK TIPS

Recognize normal labor from false labor/prodromal labor, which are characterized by **irregular contractions** that **do not cause** changes in the cervix.

+2 indicate positions **below** the ischial spines, whereas –1, –2, and –3 indicate positions **above** the ischial spines.

The Labor Process

Labor is caused by contractions that lead to cervical effacement and dilation and is organized into three stages: Stage I, Stage II, and Stage III. Stage I is the onset of labor until complete cervical dilation and usually lasts 10–12 hours in a nulliparous patient and 6–8 hours in a multiparous patient. Stage II begins when cervical dilation is complete and ends when the infant is delivered. This stage should last 2 hours in a nulliparous patient and 1 hour in a multiparous patient. Increase this limit by 1 hour in patients with an epidural. Stage III occurs once the infant is delivered and ends when the placenta is delivered.

Although many women will enter labor naturally, labor can also be induced or augmented. Induction is the process of stimulating labor with **Pitocin**, a mimetic of oxytocin that is delivered IV. Mechanical dilation or amniotomy can also be used to induce labor. Some indications for induction of labor include post-term pregnancy, PROM, IUGR, or pre-eclampsia.

Augmentation is strengthening labor. Pitocin and amniotomy can be used to augment labor, and strength of contractions can be measured using an intrauterine pressure catheter (normal readings start at 10 mm Hg and go as high as 60 mm Hg as labor progresses). The Montevideo unit is the measurement of contractions.

The status of the fetus is assessed traditionally through electronic fetal monitoring. This gives a baseline fetal heart tracing that should be within a normal range of 110–160 beats per minute (BPM). Variations from baseline should be measured; <3 variations is considered absent, 3–5 is minimal,

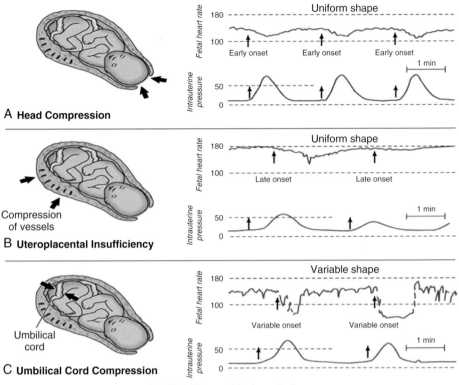

FIG. 15.4 Abnormal fetal monitoring.

5–25 is moderate, and marked is 25 BPM. Decelerations should be observed based on whether they occur early, late, or are variable. Early decelerations occur with contractions and are caused by increases in vagal tone. Late decelerations begin at peaks of contraction and return to baseline after contraction is completed and can be caused by uteroplacental insufficiency. This is the most worrying type of deceleration. Variable decelerations occur at any time and are caused by umbilical cord compression (Fig. 15.4).

During labor, you should always assess the cardinal movements: engagement, descent, flexion, internal rotation, extension, and resolution. See Fig. 15.5 for details of this process.

Three considerations for delivery are the three Ps: power, passenger, and pelvis. Problems with one or more of the three can lead to problems with delivery and may warrant C-section. For example, mismatch of passenger and pelvis can lead to cephalopelvic disproportion (CPD).

Although techniques required for vaginal delivery are not elaborated and necessary for the shelf, recognize the Ritgen maneuver, a commonly used obstetric procedure for controlling delivery of the fetal head (Fig. 15.6).

QUICK TIPS

Fetal heart monitoring can also be done from a fetal scalp electrode.

QUICK TIPS

Use fetal scalp pH to assess fetal hypoxia or acidosis by drawing blood from its scalp into a capillary tube.

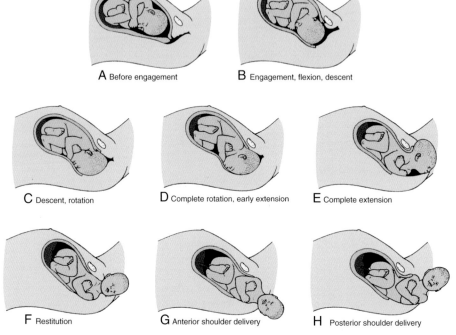

A Before engagement

B Engagement, flexion, descent

C Descent, rotation

D Complete rotation, early extension

E Complete extension

F Restitution

G Anterior shoulder delivery

H Posterior shoulder delivery

FIG. 15.5 Cardinal movements of childbirth.

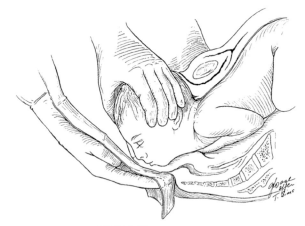

FIG. 15.6 Ritgen maneuver.

A few other procedures should be noted. An episiotomy is an incision in the perineum to facilitate delivery, and is typically medial or mediolateral. A common indication is for shoulder dystocia. Be careful to avoid extension into the rectal sphincter or rectum because this is a common complication of episiotomy (Fig. 15.7).

Vaginal delivery can also be operative through use of forceps or vacuum. For the shelf, know that forceps are

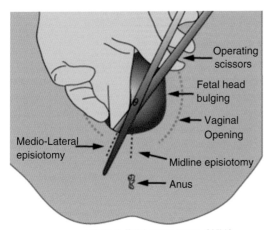

FIG. 15.7 Episiotomy types. (Wiki.)

associated with a higher rate of facial nerve palsies and perineal lacerations, whereas vacuums are associated with a higher rate of cephalohematomas and shoulder dystocias.

Finally, upon delivery of the infant, the placenta will need to be delivered. Placental separation occurs within 10 minutes of delivery but can last as long as 30 minutes—it can be recognized from cord lengthening, uterine fundal rebound, or a gush of blood. **Oxytocin is used here and is high yield for the Ob/Gyn shelf.** It is used to strengthen uterine contractions and decrease postpartum bleeding through increasing uterine muscle tone. The placenta is finally delivered by traction on the cord.

Some pharmacology to be familiar with during labor includes fentanyl, Nubain, and stadol. Morphine can be used for all patients when they present with labor. Pudendal nerve blocks are used for perianal anesthesia in patients who receive delivery via forceps or vacuum. Local anesthesia from an epidural can be used for episiotomy. General anesthesia can be used for cesarean section.

Although cesarean section (C-section) techniques are unlikely to be tested, the indications for C-sections are as follows:

- CPD
- Uterine dysfunction
- Neoplasm obstructing birth canal
- Malpresentation/position
- Previous uterine surgery
- Placenta previa
- Premature placental separation
- Umbilical prolapse

FOR THE WARDS

Epidural is done through L3-L4 catheter insertion.

Complicated Labor and Delivery

Shoulder Dystocia

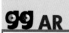
Shoulder dystocia and turtle sign

Buzz Words: Turtle sign + puffy face + facial flushing

Clinical Presentation: After head delivery, anterior shoulder cannot pass pubic symphysis. Obstetric emergency and can lead to umbilical compression. Turtle sign is the appearance and then retraction of the fetal head. Can lead to Klumpke or Erb palsy, fetal hypoxia, or cerebral palsy.

Prophylaxis (PPx): Tx diabetes, prevent obesity; age >35 = risk factor

Mechanism of Disease (MoD): N/A

Diagnostic Steps (Dx):

1. Clinical presentation

Treatment and Management Steps (Tx/Mgmt):

1. Use the **ALARMER** mnemonic:
- A = Ask for help
- L = Leg hyperflexion (McRoberts maneuver)
- A = Anterior shoulder disimpaction (pressure)
- R = Rubin maneuver
- M = Manual delivery of posterior arm
- E = Episiotomy
- R = Roll over on all fours

Complications of Cesarean Delivery

Recognize the most common complications of C-section. Obesity increases risk of ALL complications:
- Uterine infection
- Wound infection
- Thromboembolism
- Blood loss
- Uterine rupture
- Maternal death
- Injury to ureter and bladder
- Cardiopulmonary problems

Cord Compression

Buzz Words: Rapid decline to <100 BPM in fetal heart rate + decreased movement of baby

Clinical Presentation: Complications → fetal heart abnormalities, hypoxia, poor development, birth injuries

PPx: Risk factors: breech, polyhydramnios, twins, long umbilical cord

MoD: N/A

Dx:

Fetal monitoring

1. Fetal heart monitoring + clinical presentation

Tx/Mgmt:
1. Fluids and O_2
2. Change mother's position
3. Emergent C-section for emergencies
4. May need to stop contractions chemically

Cord Prolapse

Buzz Words: Severe variable decelerations + sudden decrease in fetal heart rate

Clinical Presentation: When umbilical cord comes out before presenting fetus. More common in women with amniotic sac rupture. Obstetric emergency.

PPx: N/A

MoD: N/A

Dx:
1. Fetal heart monitoring + clinical, can be considered after C-section

Tx/Mgmt:
1. Several attempts to reduce pressure and promote delivery, but most end up in C-sections

Fetal Malpresentations (Breech)

Buzz Words: Fetal head cannot be palpated on exam and baby is born bottom first

Clinical Presentation: 3%–5% of pregnant women.

PPx: N/A

MoD: Fetus does not turn to cephalic position

Dx:
1. Physical exam and pelvic ultrasound

Tx/Mgmt:
1. C-section

Preterm labor

Premature Rupture of Membranes

Buzz Words: Rupture >1 hour before labor + fluid leaks from vagina + **nitrazine blue positive fluid**

PPx: Progesterone to prevent recurrence

MoD: Not fully understood, risk factors: urinary tract infection (UTI), sexually transmitted diseases (STDs), cigarettes, drugs, hydramnios, multiple gestations, cervical insufficiency, low birth weight

Premature rupture of membranes

Dx:
1. Clinical presentation and pelvic exam
2. Ultrasound
3. Analysis of amniotic fluid with nitrazine paper (amniotic fluid will turn nitrazine paper orange to blue)

Tx/Mgmt:
1. >34 weeks → induce labor (oxytocin)

2. 24–33 weeks → waiting + steroid dose + tocolytics to prevent labor
3. <24 weeks → waiting + counseling on induction of labor

Preterm Gestation (Preterm Birth)

Buzz Words: Baby born <37 weeks

Clinical Presentation: Increased risk of CP, developmental delay, visual and hearing problems

PPx: Smoking cessation, progesterone, cervical cerclage; for threatened preterm labor, important to recognize the important role of **MgSO₄** here. Nifedipine may slow or stop labor.

MoD: Unknown, risk factors = diabetes, HTN, obesity, underweight, infections, smoking, stress, etc.

Dx:

1. Ultrasound
2. Fetal fibronectin
3. Placental alpha microglobulin

Tx/Mgmt:

1. Steroids
2. Tocolysis (NSAIDS, CCBs, B-agonists)

GUNNER PRACTICE

1. A 28-year-old, gravida 1, para 0, woman at 35 weeks' gestation comes to the physician because she is "bleeding from below." Yesterday, she noticed that there was a giant stain in her underwear that was accompanied by some episodic lower abdominal pain. During her pregnancy she smoked a pack of cigarettes every week, but was able to quit alcohol use. Glucose tolerance tests in the first trimester did not meet the threshold for gestational diabetes. A quad screen during the second trimester did not reveal any aneuploidy disorders. Her vitals are 120/80 mm Hg, 90 bpm, 98.6°F, and 14 RR. On exam, there is a pool of fluid in the vaginal canal that shows ferning and turns nitrazine paper blue. What is the most likely diagnosis?

   A. Placental abruption
   B. Placenta previa
   C. Premature rupture of membranes
   D. Vasa previa
   E. Uterine rupture

Notes

ANSWER: What Would Gunner Jess/Jim Do?

1. WWGJD? A 28 year-old, gravida 1, para 0, woman at 35 weeks' gestation comes to the physician because she is "bleeding from below." Yesterday, she noticed that there was a giant stain in her underwear that was accompanied by some episodic lower abdominal pain. During her pregnancy she smoked a pack of cigarettes every week, but was able to quit alcohol use. Glucose tolerance tests in the first trimester did not meet the threshold for gestational diabetes. Quad screen during the second trimester did not reveal any aneuploidy disorders. Her vitals are 120/80 mm Hg, 90 bpm, 98.6°F, and 14 RR. On exam, there is a pool of fluid in the vaginal canal that shows ferning and turns nitrazine paper blue. What is the most likely diagnosis?

Answer: C. Premature rupture of membranes

Explanation: One of the most straightforward disorders to identify on the Ob/Gyn shelf is premature rupture of membranes, which will present as a "pool of fluid" in the vagina that turns "nitrazine paper blue." These are clues that point to amniotic fluid leakage. There is no other condition on the shelf that would give patients this type of presentation. Because it is so straightforward, test writers will try to obscure the diagnosis by making the fluid seem as much like blood (i.e., antepartum hemorrhage) as possible. Try to ignore the distractors and zero in on the pertinent Buzz Words to answer these questions correctly.

A. Placental Abruption → Incorrect. Placental abruption is an emergency whereby the placenta detaches from the uterus, leading to bleeding in the third trimester. It would appear as blood in the vaginal canal and not as fluid.

B. Placenta previa → Incorrect. Placenta previa is painless vaginal bleeding that occurs due to a low-lying placenta. The clues here suggest amniotic fluid and not bleeding.

D. Vasa previa → Incorrect. Vasa previa is bleeding from placental vessels that overlie the cervical os. The clues here suggest amniotic fluid and not bleeding.

E. Uterine rupture → Incorrect. Uterine rupture can occur 2/2 traumatic injury or scarring from previous C-section. This would lead to massive hemorrhage.

Puerperium

Hao-Hua Wu and Leo Wang

Introduction

Puerperium (aka the postpartum period) refers to the period of time from birth to 6–8 weeks postdelivery. Disorders of the puerperium test you on the medical and psychological phenomena that can affect mothers during this time. The most high-yield concepts are the disorders that can be tested on multiple shelf exams, such as postpartum cardiomyopathy (Medicine), Sheehan syndrome (Medicine and Surgery), and postpartum blues (Psychiatry). Some high-yield disorders of the puerperium elsewhere, such as gestational trophoblastic disease/hydatidiform mole in Chapter 5 Neoplasms of the cervix, ovary, uterus, vagina and vulva and mastitis in Chapter 3 Breast Disorders.

This chapter is organized into sections on (1) Normal Postpartum Anatomic and Physiologic Changes, (2) Disorders of Lactation and Breastfeeding, (3) Puerperium Complications, and (4) Gunner Practice. Anticipate spending 5–7 hours for both the first and second pass over the course of study.

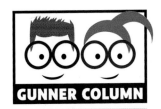

GUNNER COLUMN

Normal Postpartum Anatomic and Physiologic Changes

As mentioned in the introduction, normal postpartum anatomy and physiology will not be directly tested on the shelf. The bullet points below are concepts that may be helpful to distinguish normal from abnormal and better understand disorders of the puerperium.

- Position of uterus:
  - <24 hours postdelivery, fundus is near umbilicus
  - 1 week postdelivery, fundus is just above pubic symphysis
  - 2 weeks postdelivery, fundus is not palpable through the abdomen
  - 6–8 weeks postdelivery, uterus returns to normal size
- Normal uterus involutes (aka contracts) in the immediate postpartum period to constrict the spiral vessels in the myometrium and prevent postpartum hemorrhage (PPH).

- Normal uterus in the puerperium is nontender, firm, and smaller than expected gestation age.
  - Pathologic uteri are soft and boggy, which suggests atony or inadequate contraction.
- **Lochia** = shedding of superficial layer of basal portion of decidua 1–16 days after pregnancy
  - Normal progression of lochia coloration: Lochia rubra (red, red-brown, 1–3 days), lochia serosa (pinkish brown 2–3 weeks), lochia alba (yellowish-white)

Disorders of Lactation and Breastfeeding

Lactation is an important process of the postpartum period because it provides the mother with the ability to breastfeed her newborn. Breastfeeding helps prevent uterine atony (uterine contraction through oxytocin release), decreases incidence of ovarian cancer (less ovulation), and strengthens the newborn's immune system for 6 months (lifespan of transferred IgA) to prevent infections.

Disorders of lactation disrupt the breastfeeding process through decreased supply or inability to properly express milk supply. Examples of these include:

- Inadequate milk production from prolactinoma, previous trauma to the breast, retained placental fragments, medications (e.g., bromocriptine), and polycystic ovary syndrome
- Poor latch by baby (optimal breastfeeding position is belly to belly)

Aside from disorders of lactation, disorders of the breast can prevent breastfeeding as well. On the shelf, the most commonly tested aspect of these disorders is treatment/management (Table 16.1).

Puerperium Complications

The following complications of the puerperium specifically affect the health of the mother and are high yield on the Ob/Gyn shelf. Be sure to learn the Buzz Words and tie the concepts in with Medicine and Surgery.

Postpartum Cardiomyopathy

Buzz Words: Postpartum + symptoms/signs of heart failure (shortness of breath, orthopnea, lower extremity edema, paroxysmal nocturnal dyspnea, jugular venous distension, S3) + preeclampsia/eclampsia during pregnancy + no previous cardiomyopathy or heart failure

---

99 AR

Normal postpartum summarized UpToDate

FOR THE WARDS

Colostrum is the "breast milk" produced for the baby 2–3 days after birth that is rich in nutrients and protein (e.g., IgA)

---

99 AR

Video of Reye syndrome (and YouTube comment from a relative of Dr. Reye)

QUICK TIP

Candidiasis: 2 months after delivery + sore nipples + burning pain in breast that is worse when feeding + tips of nipples are **pink, shiny, peeling at periphery**

TABLE 16.1 Breast Feeding Problems and Treatment/Management Steps

Breast Feeding Problems	Treatment/Management
Pain General breast Nipple	*Use*: (1) Acetaminophen (enters breast milk but considered compatible), (2) short-acting NSAIDs (ibuprofen, diclofenac), (3) opiates (but observe for infant sedation) *Avoid*: Aspirin (Reye syndrome), Meperidine *Use*: Lactation consultant to optimize "latch" *Avoid*: Aspirin (ppx Reye syndrome), Meperidine
Breast engorgement	1. Self-limiting 2. Tight brassier to avoid stimulation 3. Symptom management with cool compresses, ice packs, acetaminophen/ibuprofen
Mastitis	(1) Dicloxacillin, (2) Clindamycin if methicillin-resistant *Staphylococcus aureus* (MRSA), (3) Erythromycin if allergic to penicillin, (4) continue breastfeeding with both breasts, (5) ice packs/breast binders if no breast feeding
Candidiasis	(1) Topical (e.g., clotrimazole), (2) Fluconazole, (3) treatment of newborn with Nystatin
Vasoconstriction of vasculature near nipples	(1) Warmth (e.g., wearing warm clothing, heater; think Raynaud), (2) Nifedipine

NSAIDs, Nonsteroidal anti-inflammatory drugs.

Clinical Presentation: Postpartum cardiomyopathy occurs when there is systolic heart failure in the postpartum period. Diagnosed clinically if patient has EF <45%, heart failure symptoms in postpartum period and there was no other identifiable etiology.

Prophylaxis (PPx): Avoid or treat risk factors such as pre-eclampsia/eclampsia, hypertension, multiple gestation.

Mechanism of Disease (MoD): Unknown

Diagnostic Steps (Dx):

1. H&P (S3 sound)
2. BMP/CBC and BNP (elevated)
3. CXR (enlarged heart)
4. EKG
5. Echo (EF <45%)

Treatment and Management Steps (Tx/Mgmt):

1. Treat congestive heart failure (CHF; e.g., diuretics like furosemide, salt restriction, etc.).

Postpartum Blues

Buzz Words: <2 weeks + depression symptomatology (SIGECAPS) + <4 weeks postpartum

Clinical Presentation: Postpartum blues refers to depressive symptomatology exhibited by Mom in the postpartum period that resolves **within 14 days**. It is not considered pathologic because it does not meet the 2-week threshold.

99 AR

SIGECAPS for depression symptomatology (5/9 for >2 weeks = dx of MDD): Sleep (increase/decrease), Interest loss (anhedonia), Guilt (worthlessness), Energy (low), Concentration (decreased), Appetite (decreased/increased), Psychomotor retardation, Suicidality

Those of you who have taken the Psychiatry shelf know how important timing is in making a diagnosis; identifying postpartum blues vs. postpartum depression is no different. This can affect up to half of women in the postpartum period. All you need to know for the shelf is the Buzz Words and how to differentiate from other psychiatric disorders.

PPx: Depression screening (i.e., PHQ2 or 9)

MoD: Unknown

Dx:

1. H&P, monitor for symptoms in the past 2 weeks
2. Mental Status Exam

Tx/Mgmt:

1. Rest and social support

Postpartum Depression

Buzz Words: ≥2 weeks + depression symptomatology (5/9 SIGECAPS symptoms) + <4 weeks postpartum + ambivalence toward the newborn

Clinical Presentation: Unlike postpartum blues, postpartum depression is pathologic because patients experience at least five out of nine symptoms of depression for a minimum of 2 weeks. Ambivalence to the newborn is a Buzz Word for this disorder. Screening for this disease is important to prevent suicidality and promote mother-baby bonding. Treatment in the postpartum period is the same as for any patient with depression. Care should be given as to which medications are given **intra**partum; paroxetine for instance can cause fetal cardiac defects if given during pregnancy.

PPx: Depression screening (i.e., PHQ2 or 9)

MoD: Unknown

Dx:

1. H&P, monitor for symptoms in the past 2 weeks
2. Mental status exam

Tx/Mgmt:

1. SSRIs
2. CBT
3. Admission to hospital if suicidal plan elicited

Postpartum Psychosis

Buzz Words: ≥4 weeks + within 2 weeks from birth + psychosis or manic symptoms + underlying bipolar disorder

Clinical Presentation: Patients who exhibit psychotic symptoms (e.g., audio visual hallucinations) or manic symptoms (e.g., distractibility, flight of ideas, grandiose thoughts, sleeplessness) within 2 weeks of birth and whose symptoms last for at least a month are given the diagnosis of postpartum psychosis. Having an underlying disorder, such as bipolar disorder, can predispose to this occurrence. Homicidal ideation against the newborn is considered a psychotic symptom. Learn the Buzz Words and how to differentiate from postpartum depression/blues.

PPx: None
MoD: Unknown
Dx:
1. H&P
2. Mental Status Exam
3. Urine drug test (to r/o substance use)

Tx/Mgmt:
1. Admit to hospital
2. Antipsychotic medication (e.g., risperidone)

Postpartum Hemorrhage

Buzz Words: Postpartum + vaginal bleeding + orthostatic symptoms + dizziness + pale + hypotension/tachycardia

Clinical Presentation: PPH is symptomatic bleeding from the reproductive tract in the postpartum period. PPH is an estimated blood loss of greater than or equal to 500 mL after vaginal birth, or greater than or equal to 1000 mL after Cesarean delivery. This is a frequently tested concept because it is an obstetric emergency and requires an immediate workup. However, it is important to know what to expect on the test. First, you do not need to memorize any classification systems or know the exact volume of blood lost over a period of time, although these values may be useful to know for the wards (see "Classification of postpartum hemorrhage"). Second, you will rarely be asked to identify postpartum hemorrhage because the symptoms/signs of bleeding are obvious. Thus, you will most likely be tested on the diagnostic and treatment steps to evaluate and treat postpartum hemorrhage. Uterine atony, the most common cause of postpartum hemorrhage and a high-yield Ob/Gyn shelf topic, will be presented separately. PPH can also cause many commonly tested complications, such as Sheehan syndrome, which is covered below.

PPx:
- Monitoring of vitals for signs of hemorrhage (e.g., tachycardia, tachypnea, low BP)
- Avoidance of risk factors such as preeclampsia, eclampsia, and HELLP
- Remove contained products of conception
- Take additional precautions with morbidly adherent placenta

99 AR
Causes of postpartum hemorrhage

99 AR
Classification of postpartum hemorrhage

MoD:
- Uterine atony (no contraction of myometrium)
- Laceration 2/2 trauma or surgery
- Bleeding diathesis (e.g., factor V Leiden)

Dx:
1. Pelvic exam (boggy uterus)
2. CBC to evaluate hemoglobin level
3. Coags
4. Ultrasound for echogenic mass in uterus

Tx/Mgmt:
1. Treat depending on etiology, but general workup for postpartum:
   - Oxytocin
   - Prostaglandin F2 alpha (IM to avoid bronchoconstriction)
   - If normo- or hypotensive, Methylergonovine (methergine)
   - Tamponade with Bakri balloon
   - B lynch suture
   - Uterine artery embolization (interventional radiology consult)
   - Hysterectomy

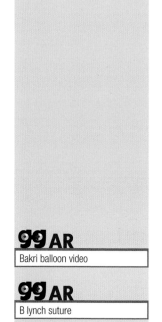

99 AR
Bakri balloon video

99 AR
B lynch suture

Uterine Atony

Buzz Words: Postpartum hemorrhage + boggy, soft uterus

Clinical Presentation: Uterine atony is defined as a state where the musculature of the uterus (myometrium) is unable to contract enough to clamp the vasculature supplying the uterus. Normal myometrium will contract, clamp, and prevent the spiral arteries of the uterus from bleeding after delivery. However, weakening of the musculature 2/2 to uterine overdistension or prolonged labor will lead to hemorrhage. For the shelf, learn the diagnostic and treatment steps well.

PPx: Avoid risk factors such as:
- Uterine overdistension (e.g., macrosomia, multiple gestation, polyhydramnios)
- Prolonged labor

MoD: Myometrium unable to contract → no muscle clamping of spiral arteries → bleeding leading to postpartum hemorrhage.

Dx:
1. Pelvic exam (boggy, soft uterus = uterine atony; small, firm uterus = no uterine atony)
2. CBC to evaluate hemoglobin levels
3. Coags
4. Ultrasound for echogenic mass in uterus

Tx/Mgmt:
1. Fluids to treat hypovolemic shock
2. Fundal/bimanual massage to stimulate uterine contraction
3. Oxytocin
4. If normo- or hypotensive, methergine (vasoconstrictor)
5. Prostaglandin F2 alpha (e.g., Carboprost)
6. Packing of bleeding with Backri balloon tamponade OR gauze OR Sengstaken-Blakemore tube
7. Uterine artery ligation (IR consult)
8. Hysterectomy

Sheehan Syndrome

Buzz Words:
- Postpartum bleeding that required aggressive resuscitation + inability to lactate + low BP + **hyponatremia** (no aldosterone)
- Inability to lactate + amenorrhea + loss of sexual hair + anorexia + weight loss + lethargy + hyponatremia + s/p delivery with postpartum hemorrhage + delayed tendon reflexes + dry skin

Clinical Presentation: Sheehan syndrome is infarction of the pituitary gland due to hemorrhage, and is frequently tested in association with postpartum hemorrhage. This is one of the most high-yield disorders because it is an Ob/Gyn topic that presents with endocrine dysfunction (e.g., hyponatremia, amenorrhea, inability to lactate), which means it is fair game for the Medicine and Surgery shelf. Thus, make sure to learn the Buzz Words, MoD, Dx, and Tx/Mgmt of this disease well. Be aware of **lymphocytic hypophysitis**, which is a cause of hypopituitarism in the postpartum period that is NOT associated with postpartum hemorrhage. On the shelf, the difference between Sheehan syndrome and lymphocytic hypophysitis is the presence or absence of hemorrhage, respectively.

PPx:
- Prevent heavy blood loss during or after delivery.
- Minimize time spent hypotensive or in need of blood transfusion.

MoD: Massive hemorrhage → pituitary hypoperfusion (pituitary is used to increase blood supply during pregnancy) → pituitary infarct/ischemic necrosis → loss of pituitary hormones

Dx:
1. Hormone levels produced by anterior pituitary gland (low FSH/LH], prolactin and TSH)
2. Progesterone ovulation challenge
3. MRI

Tx/Mgmt:
1. Hormone replacement (estrogen, progesterone, thyroid, steroids)

Uterine Inversion

Buzz Words: Postpartum period + Concomitant neoplasm (e.g., leiomyoma) + Hypovolemic shock (e.g., low BP, tachycardia) + smooth mass protruding from cervix/vagina + abdominal pain but **uterus unable to be palpated** + vaginal bleeding

Clinical Presentation: Uterine inversion is an obstetrical emergency that will frequently be tested. Typically associated with a neoplasm such as a leiomyoma. Diagnosis is purely based on clinical evidence with a "uterus that cannot be palpated from the abdomen" the defining Buzz Word. The most important thing is to stop the source of bleeding and treat the resulting hypovolemic shock. Ultrasound or imaging modalities are used for the diagnosis if and only if patient is hemodynamically stable and the diagnosis is in question.

PPx: None

MoD: Unknown

Dx:
1. Physical exam (absent fundus through transabdominal palpation; smooth mass palpated through cervix/vagina)
2. Vital signs
3. Ultrasound if hemodynamically stable

Tx/Mgmt:
1. Discontinue oxytocin or other uterotonic drugs
2. Fluids
3. Manual reduction of inverted uterus back to anatomic alignment
4. Nitroglycerin, terbutaline, magnesium sulfate, and other uterine/muscle relaxants to aid manual reduction
5. Surgical correction (e.g., laparotomy)
6. If surgical intervention impossible →hydrostatic reduction (reverse Trendelenburg and fluid applied to inverted uterus)
7. Once reduced → restart uterotonic drugs such as oxytocin to prevent further postpartum hemorrhage

Postpartum Sepsis

Buzz Words:
- Postpartum + Fever + dysuria → Postpartum infection 2/2 urinary tract infection (UTI)
- Postpartum + s/p C-section + fever + purulent drainage from incision → Postpartum infection of wound

- Postpartum infection + gray edges at perineal wound → Necrotizing fasciitis 2/2 clostridium (gray edges = necrosis; Tx with debridement and IV Abx)

Clinical Presentation: Because identifying that the patient has sepsis and the source infection is straightforward, questions about postpartum sepsis on the Ob/Gyn shelf will likely be on the diagnostic steps to r/o likely organisms. For instance, UTI and wound infection are the two most common sources of postpartum sepsis.

PPx:

- Reduce use of Foley catheterization
- IV antibiotics (i.e., ceftriaxone, clindamycin) 60 minutes before C-section surgical incision

MoD: Common causes of postpartum sepsis seen on the Ob/Gyn shelf are UTI, wound infection (e.g., surgical site for C-section, episiotomy), atelectasis, pneumonia, mastitis, endometritis.

Effect of IV antibiotics before C-sections. Cochrane review.

Dx:

1. BMP/CBC
2. UA/UCx to r/o UTI
3. Wound or blood culture
4. CXR to r/o atelectasis and pneumonia

Tx/Mgmt:

1. Antibiotics according to infection
2. Acetaminophen

Postpartum Endometritis

Buzz Words: Postpartum + fever + C-section + purulent, foul-smelling lochia + abdominal/uterine tenderness + no other sources of infection (e.g., no UTI or superficial infections)

Clinical Presentation: Endometritis in the postpartum period is defined as an infection of the endometrium of pregnancy (aka the decidua). It is a common cause of postpartum sepsis and is often associated with C-section, prior BV infection, chorioamnionitis and maternal diabetes, and colonization with Group B strep. Diagnosis is made by clinical clues. Of note, postpartum endometritis is not on the USMLE Content Outline but was added after student feedback.

PPx:

- IV Abx (i.e., ceftriaxone, clindamycin) 60 minutes before C-section surgical incision
- Avoid C-sections (biggest risk factor)

99 AR

Decidua

MoD:

- Bacterial infection 2/2 G+, G– and anaerobic organisms → spread from cervix/vagina to decidua

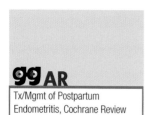

Tx/Mgmt of Postpartum
Endometritis, Cochrane Review

- Commonly associated with BV bacteria such as *Gardnerella vaginalis*

Dx: CBC (leukocytosis)

Tx/Mgmt: Clindamycin + Gentamicin

Septic Pelvic Thrombophlebitis

Buzz Words: High fever refractory to several days of antibiotic treatment + Postpartum period + r/o all other etiologies of postpartum sepsis

Clinical Presentation: Septic pelvic thrombophlebitis is a condition in which the veins in the pelvis are thrombosed and inflamed, leading to postpartum sepsis. On the shelf, this classically presents as postpartum fever or sepsis that does not resolve with antibiotic treatment. Instead, this condition will only resolve with anticoagulation. Thrombosis of the ovarian vein leads to symptoms within a week of delivery. This disorder is a diagnosis of exclusion.

PPx: None

MoD: Thrombosis of the venous system of the pelvis 2/2 endothelial damage, venous stasis, and hypercoagulable state (e.g., pregnancy); commonly thrombosis of ovarian vein. Etiology not fully understood.

Dx:
1. r/o other causes of postpartum fever (e.g., UA/UCx, BCx, examination of wound, etc.)
2. Pelvic computed tomography (CT) may show thrombosis but may not be definitive

Tx/Mgmt:
1. Heparin bridge to warfarin
2. Antibiotics

Postpartum Urinary Retention

Buzz Words: Postpartum + urinary retention + no previous bladder issues

Clinical Presentation: Postpartum urinary retention is a common disorder that occurs in the puerperium. Because the presentation is easy to identify (e.g., patient has difficulty urinating), the Buzz Words and the diagnostic steps are rarely tested. Instead, the MoD, which is a lesion to the pudendal nerve, is high-yield. Learn the MoD and move on if short on time for shelf studying. The rest of the information is included for the wards.

PPx: Avoid risk factors such as:
- Epidural anesthesia
- Episiotomy
- Instrument-assisted delivery

MoD: Injury to the pudendal nerve
Dx:
1. Pelvic exam
2. Bladder ultrasound
3. UA/UCx
Tx/Mgmt:
1. Bladder catheterization

GUNNER PRACTICE

1. After vaginal delivery 20 hours ago, a 30-year-old, gravida 2, para 2, woman presents with a fever. She denies dysuria, urinary frequency, or urgency. Her vital signs are 101°F, 99 bpm, 20 RR, 110/78 mm Hg, and 89% on room air. An exam shows reddish fluid around the vaginal canal, and a non-tender firm uterus the same size as week 20 of gestation. Her heart rate and rhythm are regular and there are no murmurs, rubs, or gallops, and her lungs have decreased breath sounds bilaterally. Episiotomy site is clean, dry, and intact. Labs are ordered and urine is drawn with a Foley catheter. What is the most likely diagnosis?
   A. Septic pelvic thrombophlebitis
   B. Endometritis
   C. Atelectasis
   D. Urinary tract infection
   E. Normal postpartum state

2. Forty-eight hours after C-section, a 28-year-old, gravida 1, para 1, woman presents with abdominal pain. She reports nausea and two episodes of nonbloody, nonbilious emesis, but no urinary frequency or urgency. Her vital signs are 100.4°F, 99 bpm, 20 RR, 120/85 mm Hg, and 95% on room air. Exam shows tenderness to palpation of the right and left lower quadrant of the abdomen, yellowish fluid around the vaginal canal, and a firm but tender uterus. A complete blood count shows a white cell count of 16,000/mm^3 and a urinalysis positive for RBCs. What is the next best step in management of the patient's pain?
   A. Heparin
   B. Dilatation and curettage
   C. Uterine artery embolization
   D. Fluids
   E. IV clindamycin and gentamicin

3. Twelve hours after a vaginal delivery assisted by episiotomy, a 29-year-old woman, gravida 2, para 2, presents with vaginal bleeding and shortness of breath. No

complications were reported during the delivery and the entire placenta had been eased out of the vaginal canal after 15 minutes of gentle traction on the umbilical cord. The episiotomy site appears to be clean, dry, and intact. The patient's vitals are 99.5°F, 100 bpm, 20 RR, 70/40 mm Hg, and 91% on room air. On the abdominal exam, there is no tenderness of the right and left lower quadrants, but the uterus cannot be palpated. Patient is started on fluids and labs are ordered. What is the most likely diagnosis?

A. Uterine atony
B. Uterine inversion
C. Endometritis
D. Placenta accrete
E. Sheehan syndrome

NOTES

ANSWERS: What Would Gunner Jess/Jim Do?

1. WWGJD? After vaginal delivery 20 hours ago, a 30-year-old, gravida 2, para 2, woman presents with a fever. She denies dysuria, urinary frequency, or urgency. Her vital signs are **101°F**, 99 bpm, 20 RR, 110/78 mm Hg, and **89% on room air.** An exam shows reddish fluid around the vaginal canal, and a non-tender firm uterus the same size as week 20 of gestation. Her heart rate and rhythm are regular and there are no murmurs, rubs or gallops, and her lungs have **decreased breath sounds bilaterally. Incision site is clean, dry, and intact.** Labs are ordered and urine is drawn with a Foley catheter. **What is the most likely diagnosis?**

Answer: C. Atelectasis

Explanation: This patient has postpartum fever due to atelectasis, which is the most common cause of postoperative fever in the first 24 hours (something that is frequently emphasized in the Surgery shelf but may be less commonly mentioned in Ob/Gyn study resources). Clues that support atelectasis are the decreased O_2 sat and the decreased breath sounds bilaterally. Other more common causes of infection, such as UTI and wound infection, were less likely given the lack of symptoms.

A. Septic pelvic thrombophlebitis (SPT) → Incorrect. The classic presentation of SPT is fever refractory to antibiotic treatment. Typically SPT, which is a thrombosis of the pelvic veins, is seen a few days after delivery and not within the 24-hour mark.

B. Endometritis → Incorrect. Although a common cause of postpartum fever and associated with C-sections, endometritis is unlikely here due to a lack of key Buzz Words, such as "purulent" or "foul-smelling" lochia. The reddish fluid described in the question stem is likely lochia rubra.

D. Urinary tract infection → Incorrect. There are no signs or symptoms pointing to a UTI. Diagnostic steps for UTI would have been to get a UA and UCx from urine out of the catheter. Patient likely needed a Foley catheter because of postpartum urinary retention, a common phenomenon in the puerperium.

E. Normal postpartum state → Incorrect. Patients who have a fever (e.g., >100.4°F) with concomitant symptoms (e.g., decreased breath sounds, decreased O_2 sat) likely have a developing or ongoing infection. There are some states that can cause an elevated temperature without an infectious source, such as breast engorgement, but the pulmonary source was clearly indicated in the question stem.

2. WWGJD? Forty-eight hours after C-section, a 28-year-old, gravida 1, para 1, woman presents with abdominal pain. She reports feeling nauseous and two episodes of nonbloody, nonbilious emesis, but no urinary frequency or urgency. Her vital signs are 100.4°F, 99 bpm, 20 RR, 120/85 mm Hg, and 95% on room air. Exam shows tenderness to palpation of the right and left lower quadrant of the abdomen, a smelly, yellowish fluid around the vaginal canal, and a firm but tender uterus. A complete blood count showed a white cell count of 16,000/mm³ and a urinalysis positive for RBCs. What is the next best step in management of the patient's pain?

Answer: E. IV clindamycin and gentamicin

Explanation: The patient has endometritis, which is one of the most common causes of postpartum fever and is the result of cervicovaginal bacteria that gets transported to the uterus. The Buzz Word for endometritis is a smelly, purulent lochia, and the most appropriate first treatment for this is clindamycin and gentamicin given intravenously.

A. Heparin → Incorrect. This would be the treatment of choice for patients with septic pelvic thrombophlebitis, which is seen with postpartum fever refractory to antibiotics.

B. Dilatation and curettage → Incorrect. This would be the correct treatment for postpartum hemorrhage caused by retention of products of conception.

C. Uterine artery embolization → Incorrect. This would be the correct treatment for a patient with postpartum hemorrhage refractory to pharmacologic intervention and tamponade by Bakri balloon.

D. Fluids → Incorrect. Patient does not appear to be bleeding and blood pressure appears normotensive.

3. WWGJD? Twelve hours after a vaginal delivery assisted by episiotomy, a 29-year-old woman, gravida 2, para 2, presents with vaginal bleeding and shortness of breath. No complications were reported during the delivery and the entire placenta had been eased out of the vaginal canal after 15 minutes of gentle traction on the umbilical cord. The episiotomy site appears to be clean, dry and intact. Patients vitals are 99.5°F, 100 bpm, 20 RR, 70/40 mm Hg,

91% on RA. On the abdominal exam, there is no tenderness of the right and left lower quadrants, but **the uterus cannot be palpated.** Patient is started on fluids and labs are ordered. **What is the most likely diagnosis?**

Answer: B. Uterine inversion

Explanation: Three key Buzz Words indicate that this patient has uterine inversion, which is an obstetric emergency. First, this is a question about the postpartum period, as indicated by the first sentence. Second, the patient underwent a long period of traction with the umbilical cord, which is a risk factor for inverting the uterus into the vaginal canal. Third, the uterus cannot be palpated on the abdomen, when it can usually be felt above the level of the pubic symphysis. Thus, it is important to reduce the uterus into anatomic position by manual pressure, surgical means, or hydrostatic pressure.

A. Uterine atony → Incorrect. Although uterine atony is a common cause of vaginal bleeding, the fact that the examiner could not feel the uterus meant that this was more likely uterine inversion.

C. Endometritis → Incorrect. Endometritis is caused by an infection of the decidua and can lead to septic shock. However, it is less likely to present with vaginal bleeding.

D. Placenta accreta → Incorrect. Placenta accreta is a condition where the chorionic villi of the placenta have an abnormal attachment to the myometrium rather than decidua basalis. It is part of a spectrum of disorders (Placenta increta = chorionic villi that invades the myometrium; Placenta percreta = chorionic villi that attached proximal to the myometrium) that lead to the placenta being abnormally stuck in place after birth. This leads to postpartum hemorrhage, because the placenta bleeds. Treatment for this is dilatation and curettage, methotrexate, arterial ligation, or hysterectomy. However, this answer choice is much less likely because it was stated that the placenta was delivered from the vaginal canal.

E. Sheehan syndrome → Incorrect. Sheehan syndrome is an infarct of the pituitary gland that occurs as a result of excessive postpartum hemorrhage. Thus, this patient could have eventually had Sheehan syndrome as manifested by various pituitary hormone deficiencies. However, no endocrine abnormalities means that the patient is unlikely to have reached that stage yet.

99 AR

Placenta accreta ACOG
Committee Opinion

Disorders of the Newborn

Hao-Hua Wu and Leo Wang

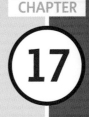

Introduction

The disorders covered in this chapter are very diverse and are grouped by organizing principles (i.e., amenorrhea, aneuploidy, traumatic, etc.). Expect at least five questions on the Ob/Gyn shelf from this chapter's material, the most high-yield being the disorders of ambiguous genitalia and disorders identified on the Quad screen.

This chapter is divided into (1) Amenorrhea and Ambiguous Genitalia, (2) Aneuploidy Disorders, (3) Traumatic Disorders, (4) Infections, (5) Miscellaneous, and (6) Gunner Practice. Anticipate spending 4–8 hours perusing the material and completing the questions.

Amenorrhea and Ambiguous Genitalia

Androgen Insensitivity Syndrome

Buzz Words: No hair + female phenotype + no uterus/fallopian tube/ovary + bilateral inguinal masses + blind vaginal pouch + 46XY + primary amenorrhea + breast development with no hair

Clinical Presentation: Androgen insensitivity syndrome (AIS) has end-organ resistance to androgens because of a mutated androgen receptor. Patients have functioning testes that secrete anti-müllerian hormone, which is why there are no müllerian structures (e.g., no uterus, fallopian tube, or ovary). However, there is a blind vaginal pouch because of no androgen stimulation. The most important Buzz Words for AIS are patients with no hair and XY chromosome.

Prophylaxis (PPx): N/A

Mechanism of Disease (MoD): Dysfunction of androgen receptors → free floating testosterone converted to estrogen → feminization of external genitalia and breast development

Diagnostic Steps (Dx):

1. No pubic or axillary hair, no penis/scrotum on physical exam
2. Karyotype analysis (46XY)
3. Abdominal ultrasound (finds **cryptorchid testes**)

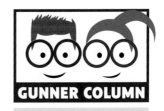

GUNNER COLUMN

Treatment and Management Steps (Tx/Mgmt):

1. Gonadectomy **after puberty** to reduce chance of testicular carcinoma
2. Estrogen therapy after removal of gonads

5-Alpha Reductase Deficiency

Buzz Words: 46XY + Amenorrhea + **ambiguous external
genitalia until puberty** + male internal genitalia (seminal
vesicles, epididymis, ejaculatory duct, ductus deferens)

Clinical Presentation: 5-alpha reductase converts testosterone to dihydrotestosterone (DHT). Patients who have a
deficiency of 5-alpha reductase cannot produce DHT,
leading to disruption in the formation of the male external genitalia. The result is ambiguous genitalia, although
many newborns can appear to have female genitalia
(thus, the reason this is tested on the Ob/Gyn shelf).
The hallmark of this disease is that male sexual characteristics start to develop during puberty, coinciding with
a normal surge of hormone production.

PPx: N/A

MoD: Mutation of the *SRD5A2* gene for 5-alpha reductase
deficiency

Dx:

1. Physical exam
2. Karyotype analysis
3. Abdominal ultrasound

Tx/Mgmt:

1. Hormone replacement therapy
2. Gonadectomy if female gender assignment

Aromatase Deficiency

Buzz Words:

- **46XX** + Normal internal genitalia (uterus, fallopian
  tube, ovary) + **ambiguous external genitalia** + primary
  amenorrhea + clitoromegaly + sexual infantilism + high
  testosterone/androstenedione + high follicle-stimulating
  hormone/luteinizing hormone (FSH/LH) + low estrogen +
  multiple ovarian cysts (e.g., multicystic ovaries) → aromatase deficiency
- **Masculinization of mother during pregnancy** +
  masculinization resolves with delivery → aromatase
  deficiency of baby

Clinical Presentation: Aromatase converts testosterone into
estrogen. Patients with aromatase deficiency can be
either XX or XY. On the Ob/Gyn shelf, you will only be
tested on the 46XX patients. You will get one of two
chief complaints: (1) newborn with ambiguous genitalia

with eventual primary amenorrhea and multiple ovarian cysts, or (2) a mother who experiences virilization during pregnancy. In both cases, the symptoms are caused by high testosterone levels. Treatment for 46XX patients is hormone therapy to replace the missing estrogen.

PPx: N/A

MoD: Mutation of the *CYP919A1* gene

Dx:

1. FSH/LH (high)
2. Estrogen (low)
3. Testosterone and androstenedione concentrations (high)
4. Pelvic ultrasound → Ovarian cysts

Tx/Mgmt:

1. Estrogen replacement

Congenital Adrenal Hyperplasia

Buzz Words:

- 46XX + ambiguous genitalia or phallus/scrotum present + virilization + hypotension + hyperaldosterone + increased sex steroid→ 21-alpha hydroxylase
- 46XX + delayed puberty, no ambiguous genitalia + hypertension → 17-alpha hydroxylase deficiency
- 46XX + ambiguous genitalia + virilization + high levels of sex hormones + hypertension → 11-beta hydroxylase

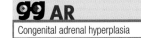
Congenital adrenal hyperplasia

Clinical Presentation: Congenital adrenal hyperplasia consists of three types of disorders that do not make cortisol, which is what induces the hyperplasia of the adrenal glands. Depending on the enzyme deficiency, however, different steroids are high or low.

- **21-alpha hydroxylase deficiency** = decreased mineralocorticoid → hypotension + ambiguous genitalia
  - Can be salt wasting (e.g., no aldosterone, no salt retention → hyponatremia and hyperkalemia) or virilizing (aldosterone is present; only cortisol synthesis is impaired)
- **17-hydroxylase deficiency** = mineralocorticoid producing → hypertension + delayed puberty + androgens not elevated so no ambiguous genitalia
- **11-beta hydroxylase deficiency** = mineralocorticoid-producing (11-deoxycorticosterone) → hypertension + ambiguous genitalia

PPx: N/A

MoD:

- For 21-hydroxylase deficiency, there is no conversion of progesterone to deoxycorticosterone (intermediates on aldosterone pathway) and 17-hydroxyprogesterone to 11-deoxycortisol (on the cortisol pathway → buildup of hormone precursors that are converted to androgens → ambiguous genitalia for 46XX.

- For 17-hydroxylase deficiency → progesterone and pregnenolone are not converted to 17-hydroxyprogresterone and 17-hydroxypregnenolone, respectively → no production of cortisol and buildup of aldosterone/androgen.
- For 11-beta hydroxylase deficiency → penultimate step of aldosterone (deoxycorticosterone to corticosterone) and terminal step of cortisol (11-deoxycortisol → cortisol) pathways are inhibited → even though no aldosterone, 11-deoxycortisol acts as weak mineralocorticoid → shunts hormones to androgens → ambiguous genitalia.

Dx:
1. Physical exam
2. Ultrasound to identify internal genitalia
3. Labs for sex steroids (e.g., elevated androgens in 21-and 11-hydroxylase deficiency)
4. Karyotype

Tx/Mgmt:
1. Glucocorticoids for all types of CAH
2. If 21-alpha hydroxylase deficiency → mineralocorticoid
3. If 17-hydroxylase → sex steroids (estrogen)

XY Gonadal Dysgenesis (Swyer Syndrome)

Buzz Words: 46XY + internal/external female genitalia + nonfunctional ovaries + axillary/pubic hair present

Clinical Presentation: XY gonadal dysgenesis (aka Swyer syndrome) is the only disorder that has a 46XY karyotype and **both** internal and external female reproductive structures. This is because of a defect in the *SRY* gene, thus stunting testicular formation

PPx: N/A

MoD: *SRY* gene defect in Y chromosome → no testicular formation → no testosterone or anti müllerian hormone produced → Wolffian ducts fail to develop and müllerian ducts take their place.

Dx:
1. FSH/LH (high, no estrogen downregulating them)
2. Karyotype

Tx/Mgmt:
1. **Immediate** removal of gonads (don't wait until puberty).
2. Hormone replacement (estrogen for breast development; progestin for periods).
3. Embryo transfer if patient wishes to be pregnant.

QUICK TIPS

Do not confuse XY gonadal dysgenesis with XY disorder of sex development (DSD), which is a 46XX individual with male external genitalia {2/2} excessive exposure to androgens as a neonate. Congenital adrenal hyperplasia is an example of XY DSD.

QUICK TIPS

Swyer syndrome requires immediate removal of gonads because risk of cancer is much higher than in AIS, in which gonads can be removed after puberty.

TABLE 17.1 Quad Screen Results

Quad Screen Results	AFP	hCG	Inhibin A	Estriol
Down syndrome	Decreased	Increased	Increased	Decreased
Edward syndrome	Decreased	Decreased	Normal	Decreased
Turner syndrome	Decreased	Decreased (increased with hydrops fetalis)	Decreased	Decreased (increased with hydrops fetalis)

AFP, Alpha fetoprotein; *hCG*, human chorionic gonadotropin.

Aneuploidy Disorders

Aneuploidy disorders are caused by an abnormal number of chromosomes. These are high-yield on the Ob/Gyn shelf because they are screened for at 15–20 weeks gestation with the Quad screen, which measures four variables:

- Alpha fetoprotein (AFP, increased in neural tube defects, decreased in trisomy 21 and 18)
- Estriol
- Beta-human chorionic gonadotropin (hCG)
- Inhibin A

Depending on the levels of these four measurements, one can ascertain one of four aneuploidy disorders: Down syndrome (trisomy 21), Edward syndrome (trisomy 18), Patau syndrome (trisomy 13), and Turner syndrome (XO) (Table 17.1).

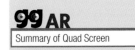
Summary of Quad Screen

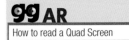
How to read a Quad Screen

Down Syndrome

Buzz Words:
- Newborn **+ sandal gap toes** + hypotonia + flattened nasal bridge + small, rotated, cup-shaped ears + small size + **Simian creases** + epicanthic folds + oblique palpebral fissures
- High inhibin A + **high hCG** + low Estriol and **low AFP**

Clinical Presentation: Down syndrome (aka trisomy 21) is the constellation of signs and symptoms that occur {2/2} presence of three copies of chromosome 21. The most high-yield Buzz Words are sandal gap toes and simian crease of the hands. This is very frequently tested on the shelf exam and is seen in Pediatrics, Medicine, Surgery, Neurology, and Psychiatry. For the Ob/Gyn shelf, just be able to identify the newborn Buzz Words. You will not be tested on the medical complications of Down syndrome that occur after the newborn period (e.g., increased risk of Alzheimer disease, risk of ALL, atlantoaxial instability, etc.). However, be aware of the **cardiac** and **GI** signs that can present at birth:
- Ventricular septal defect (e.g., "holosystolic murmur")
- Atrial septal defects (e.g., "fixed split S2" and "low-grade diastolic murmur")

- Endocardial defects
- Hirschsprung disease (e.g., "failure to pass meconium")
- Intestinal atresia
- Annular pancreas
- Imperforate anus

PPx:

- First trimester: Pregnancy-associated protein A (PAPP-A) and free beta hCG (known as the combined test) = screening against Down syndrome; positive if **high hCG** and low PAPP-A
- First trimester: Nuchal translucency and presence/absence of nasal bone on ultrasound = screening against Down syndrome
- Second semester: Quad screening test; avoid pregnancy during advanced maternal age

MoD: Nondisjunction of chromosome 21 → trisomy 21

Dx:

1. Karyotype analysis with amniocentesis if Quad screening shows decreased AFP/estriol and increased hCG and inhibin A
2. Echo for cardiac defects
3. Abdominal ultrasound for abdominal defects

Tx/Mgmt:

1. Supportive
2. Surgery to repair cardiac or abdominal defects

Edward Syndrome (Trisomy 18)

Buzz Words: Low estriol, hCG, AFP + normal/low inhibin A on Quad screen

Rocker-bottom feet + VSD + overlapping flexed fingers + horseshoe kidney → Trisomy 18

Clinical Presentation: Trisomy 18 is aneuploidy of chromosome 18 that causes rocker-bottom feet, horseshoe kidney, and VSD. It is one of the aneuploidy disorders screened for in the Quad screen and can be remembered by having all low (except for inhibin A) levels on the four serum markers.

PPx: Quad screen test

MoD: Nondisjunction of chromosome 18

Dx:

1. If Quad screen positive, karyotype with amniocentesis

Tx/Mgmt:

1. Surgery for VSD

Patau Syndrome (Trisomy 13)

Buzz Words: Newborn + cleft lip + polydactyly

Clinical Presentation: Trisomy 13 is aneuploidy of chromosome 13, which causes cleft lip and polydactyly of the newborn. Signs and symptoms can be remembered by turning "13" 90 degrees to its side.

PPx: N/A

MoD: Nondisjunction of chromosome 13

Dx:

1. If Quad screen positive, karyotype with amniocentesis

Tx/Mgmt:

1. Surgery to correct cleft palate

Turner Syndrome

Buzz Words:

- Amenorrhea + infertility + streak ovaries + short stature + coarctation of aorta (differences in BP among extremities) + webbed neck + cubitus valgus (when forearm is angled away from body to greater degree than normal when fully extended) + bicuspid aortic valve + horseshoe kidney + low hairline (where hair starts growing is too close to eyebrows) + **osteoporosis** (2/2 ovarian dysgenesis) + lymphedema

- **Stem clues for Noonan syndrome:** Widely spaced nipples + dyslexia + amenorrhea + short + sexual immaturity + **face tapers from forehead to chin** + thickened neck + normal genotype (hard to differentiate, except for bilateral deficit)

Clinical Presentation: Turner syndrome is high yield on the shelf. For the Ob/Gyn shelf, you will not be tested on the Quad screen results of Turner syndrome; rather you will be presented with Buzz Words. It affects only females; XO on chromosomal analysis can present in many different ways: newborns may have lower than normal blood pressure in their lower extremities (coarctation of aorta), toddlers may have a webbed neck and grow to below average in height, teenagers have amenorrhea (from streak ovaries), and adults may have cardiovascular problems due to a bicuspid aortic valve. Patients with Turner syndrome have **normal cognitive abilities.** Make sure to learn the Buzz Words, MoD, Dx, and Tx/Mgmt of this disease well because it can also appear on your Pediatrics, Ob/Gyn, and Medicine shelf.

PPx: N/A

MoD: XO genotype:

- Rib notching 2/2 development of collateral vessels that develop to bypass coarctation of aorta

- Lymphedema occurs 2/2 dysgenesis of the lymphatic network

99 AR

Buzz Word mnemonic for Patau syndrome

QUICK TIPS

In males, the equivalent is Noonan syndrome, except the buzz word is cubitus valgus.

QUICK TIPS

Continuous murmur throughout chest + rib notching on chest x-ray = coarctation of the aorta

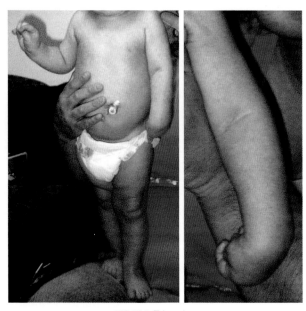

FIG. 17.1 Erb palsy.

Dx:
1. FSH levels (will likely have high FSH and LH because of ovarian dysgenesis and no negative feedback)
2. Inhibin levels (will likely be low because inhibin → measure of ovarian function)
3. Estrogen/testosterone → lower estrogen and normal testosterone
4. **Karyotpe analysis for definitive diagnosis**
5. ECG and echo to screen for cardiac abnormalities
6. BMP to look at renal function

Tx/Mgmt:
1. Treatment for coarctation of the aorta (e.g., indomethacin) and bicuspid aortic valve (e.g., valvular replacement)
2. Recombinant human growth hormone

Traumatic Disorders of the Newborn

Erb-Duchenne Palsy (Upper Trunk Lesion)

Buzz Words: Recently delivered infant + arm adducted, pronated, wrist flexed (Fig. 17.1)

Clinical Presentation: Erb palsy is a lesion of the upper trunk that can be caused by obstetrical-related brachial nerve trauma or traumatic injury as an adult. For the Surgery shelf, it is more likely you'll see this in the setting of newborns because surgical management can be more successful for refractory cases. Patients with Erb palsy present with the

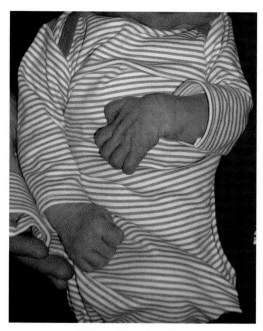

FIG. 17.2 Klumpke palsy.

"Waiter's Tip" or "Bellman's" posture. If severe enough, can be associated with T1 avulsion and Horner syndrome.

PPx: Avoid shoulder dystocia

MoD: Traction on upper trunk (C5-C6) of brachial plexus 2/2 shoulder dystocia → weakness of deltoid, biceps, infraspinatus, wrist extensors

Dx:
1. Clinical presentation

Tx/Mgmt:
1. Conservative (gentle massage, physical therapy)
2. If T1 avulsion, Horner syndrome or no resolution of symptoms, neuroma excision and interpositional nerve grafting

Review of nerve transfer indications in obstetrical brachial plexus palsy

Klumpke Palsy (Brachial Plexus Lower Trunk Injury)

Buzz Words:
- Adult + grabbed branch during fall + atrophy of hypothenar muscles + sensory loss of pinky and lateral ring finger → Klumpke palsy 2/2 mechanical stress
- Recent delivered infant subjected to upward force on arm during delivery + absent grasp reflex + claw hand → Klumpke palsy 2/2 birth trauma (Fig. 17.2)

Clinical Presentation: Klumpke palsy is a lesion of the lower trunk that can be caused by obstetrical-related brachial nerve trauma or traumatic injury as an adult. For the

Surgery shelf, it is more likely you'll see this in the setting of newborns because surgical management can be more successful for refractory cases. Characterized by claw hand. If severe enough, can be associated with T1 avulsion and Horner syndrome.

PPx: Avoid stretch-like motions or shoulder dystocias

MoD: Traction on lower trunk (C8-T1) of brachial plexus {2/2} shoulder dystocia→ weakness of intrinsic hand muscles: Lumbricals, interossei, thenar, hypothenar, sensory loss of ulnar distribution → extended wrist + hyperextended metacarpophalangeal (MCP) joints + fixed interphalangeal joints + absent grasp reflex.

Dx:
1. Clinical exam

Tx/Mgmt:
1. Conservative (gentle massage, physical therapy)
2. If T1 avulsion, Horner syndrome or no resolution of symptoms, neuroma excision and interpositional nerve grafting

Congenital Infections

You may be asked to identify a congenital infection on the Ob/Gyn shelf. The following are the seven most common ones tested. Be sure to know the difference between early and late congenital syphilis (<2 years old vs. ≥2 years old) as well what periventricular vs. intracranial calcifications mean (former = congenital CMV; latter = congenital toxoplasmosis). PPx, MoD, Dx, and Tx/Mgmt are unlikely to be tested on the Ob/Gyn shelf and will be covered in Pediatrics (Table 17.2).

Miscellaneous Disorders of the Newborn

Kallman Syndrome

Buzz Words: **Anosmia** + short stature + small genitals + amenorrhea + no hair + no breast development + delayed puberty

Clinical Presentation: Kallman syndrome is a disorder of neuron migration that leads to **anosmia** and **hypogonadism.** No other condition in the shelf exams has this combination of Buzz Words. Remember this well, because it can appear on the Pediatrics and Medicine shelf exams as well.

PPx: N/A

MoD: Failure of fetal GnRH and olfactory neurons to migrate → rhinencephalon hypoplasia (no smell) and hypogonadotropic hypogonadism (no functional ovaries)

TABLE 17.2 Congenital Infections

Buzz Words	Infection
Newborn + failure to thrive + lymphadenopathy + thrush + maternal IV drug use	Congenital human immunodeficiency virus
Newborn + sensorineural hearing loss + patent ductus arteriosus murmur + cataracts (leukocoria) or glaucoma + hepatosplenomegaly + thrombocytopenic purpura (blueberry muffin rash)	Congenital rubella
Newborn + sensorineural hearing loss + no heart abnormality + **periventricular** calcifications + hepatosplenomegaly + chorioretinitis + microcephaly	Congenital *Cytomegalovirus*
≥2 years old + **sensorineural hearing loss** + no heart abnormality + saber shins + frontal bossing + **interstitial keratitis** + **Hutchinson incisors** + bulldog facies {2/2} maldevelopment of maxilla + gummatous ulcers of nose and hard palate	Late congenital syphilis (≥2 years old)
<2 year old + runny nose + copper-colored macular rash on palms and soles + vesiculobullous eruptions + hepatosplenomegaly	Early congenital syphilis (<2 years old)
Newborn + microcephaly + limb hypoplasia + intrauterine growth restriction + cataracts + mother with pruritic vesicular rash	Congenital varicella syndrome
Newborn + **intracranial** calcifications + chorioretinitis + hydrocephalus + hepatosplenomegaly	Congenital toxoplasmosis

Dx:
1. FSH/LH (low, indicating GnRH deficiency)

Tx/Mgmt:
1. Estrogen and progesterone to develop sex characteristics, build bone and muscle, and improve fertility
2. Pulsatile GnRH

Gastroschisis and Omphalocele

Buzz Words: Newborn + abdominal organs with no covering → gastroschisis

Newborn + abdominal organs with covering membrane → omphalocele

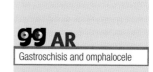

Gastroschisis and omphalocele

Clinical Presentation: Gastroschisis and omphalocele are abdominal wall defects that are seen at birth. One has no abdominal membrane covering (gastroschisis) while the other one does (omphalocele). On the Ob/Gyn shelf, only the Buzz Words will be tested.

PPx: N/A

MoD: N/A

Dx:
1. Physical exam
2. Ultrasound

Tx/Mgmt:
1. Surgery

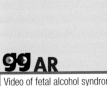

MNEMONIC

CATCH DiGeorge if you can
(**C**onotruncal cardiac defects,
Abnormal facies, **T**hymic
aplasia/hypoplasia, **C**left palate,
Hypocalcemia)

Fetal Alcohol Syndrome

Buzz Words: Smooth philtrum + attention-deficit/hyperactivity disorder (ADHD)-like symptoms + Microcephaly + Mental retardation (most common acquired cause)

Clinical Presentation: Fetal alcohol syndrome (FAS) is the constellation of signs and symptoms that occur to the fetus 2/2 alcohol use during pregnancy. The most characteristic Buzz Word for FAS is smooth philtrum of the upper lip. The mechanism is unknown and treatment is supportive.

PPx: Avoid alcohol during pregnancy

MoD: Unknown

Dx:
1. Physical exam
2. Ultrasound

Tx/Mgmt:
1. Supportive
2. Counseling

22q11.2 Deletion Syndrome (DiGeorge Syndrome, Velocardiofacial Syndrome, Conotruncal Anomaly Face Syndrome)

Buzz Words: Conotruncal cardiac defects (cyanotic disorders such as truncus arteriosus and Tetralogy of Fallot) + Abnormal facies (low set ears and micrognathia) + Thymic aplasia/hypoplasia + Cleft palate + Hypocalcemia (seizures, QT prolongation)

Clinical Presentation: 22q11.2 deletion syndrome is a genetic disorder that describes the phenotypical traits of a patient with a deletion at 22q11.2, which is the most common microdeletion in humans. This was formerly known as DiGeorge syndrome, velocardiofacial syndrome, or conotruncal anomaly face syndrome, but was changed into a unifying name once it was clear the genetic abnormality was the same. Because many of the shelf questions were written a while ago, you may still see the terms DiGeorge syndrome or velocardiofacial syndrome pop up. Just be sure to know the distinguishing features of this syndrome: low-set ears, micrognathia, conotruncal abnormalities (e.g., Tetralogy of Fallot, truncus arteriosus), immunodeficiency aplasia/hypoplasia, cleft palate, and hypocalcemia.

One thing to be aware of is that the shelf presentation of 22q11.2 deletion syndrome could be very different from what you see clinically. Many patients with 22q11.2 deletion syndrome are now living into adulthood and have been found to suffer from concomitant psychiatric

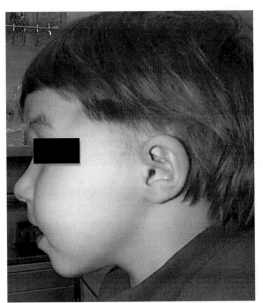

FIG. 17.3 Characteristic faces of 22q11.2 deletion syndrome including micrognathia and low-set ears.

disease (e.g., schizophrenia), intellectual disability, autoimmune disorders, hypothyroidism, Parkinson disease, and neurodegenerative disease. These manifestations have not been classically seen on the shelf as Buzz Words for 22q11.2 deletion syndrome (aka DiGeorge aka velocardiofacial syndrome). However, as questions are updated, these adult manifestations may begin to appear as well.

PPx: Patients with DiGeorge should avoid live vaccines such as rotavirus, yellow fever, polio because of thymic aplasia → immunodeficiency; inactivated or killed vaccines are OK.

MoD: Chromosome 22q11.2 deletion → defective development of pharyngeal pouches hypocalcemia 2/2 hypoplasia of parathyroid glands + cleft palate + congenital heart disease (truncus arteriosus) + immunodeficiency 2/2 thymic aplasia/hypoplasia and resultant T-cell deficiency.

Dx:
1. BMP to assess for life-threatening hypocalcemia
2. Chest x-ray (CXR) will show absent thymus
3. ECG and echo to assess cardiac defects
4. Chromosomal analysis

Tx/Mgmt:
1. Replete calcium if hypocalcemic
2. Surgical correction of conotruncal cardiac defects
3. Surgical correction of cleft palate
4. Genetic counseling (Fig. 17.3)

Management of 22q11.2 Deletion Syndrome

GUNNER PRACTICE

1. A 16-year-old girl comes into the doctor's office due to amenorrhea concerns. Her parents are worried that she has not yet had her period, even though her two sisters had menstrual cycles at the age of 13. The patient is self-conscious because her friends make fun of her for not having any breast development. She thinks this is why she has never had a boyfriend. When the parents step out of the room, the girl states that she has never been sexually active and does not take any medications. On exam, she is fifth percentile for her age in height and has Tanner stage 1 breast development. There is a 2/6 holosystolic murmur that can be heard in the midsternal border. Her physical exam is otherwise normal. A urine pregnancy test is negative. What is the next best step in diagnosis?
   A. Transvaginal ultrasound
   B. Transabdominal ultrasound
   C. Follicle-stimulating hormone level
   D. Complete blood count
   E. Karyotype analysis

2. A 16-year-old girl comes into the doctor's office because of her parents' concern about amenorrhea. Her mother had her period when she was 12 years old and is concerned that her daughter is not developing as quickly. The patient is less concerned and states that she feels great. Unlike her friends, she does not have to shave and never needs tampons. Her breast development is Tanner stage 3. Her physical exam reveals a short vaginal pouch with no palpable uterus or adnexa. Karyotype analysis shows 46XY. What is the most likely mechanism for her amenorrhea?
   A. Deficiency of 17-alpha hydroxylase
   B. Defect in the *SRY* gene
   C. 5-alpha reductase deficiency
   D. Defect of an androgen receptor
   E. Deficiency of 21-alpha hydroxylase

3. A 34-year-old, gravida 3, para 2, woman who is 17 weeks pregnant comes to the physician for a prenatal visit. During her visit she states that the swelling in her hands and feet are unchanged from the last time she was seen. She gets very tired at times during the day but is still able to complete her tasks at work. Last weekend, she accidentally had one sip of wine, but has not had any alcohol since the beginning of her pregnancy. The only medication she takes right now are folate supplements. She is still sexually active with her husband. Her vitals are 120/80 mm Hg, 90 bpm, 98.6°F,

and 14 RR. Her uterus is enlarged. Fetal heart rate is within normal limits. Her Quad screen results are as follows:

Alpha fetoprotein: Decreased

Inhibin A: Increased

hCG: Increased

Estriol: Decreased

What is the most likely diagnosis of the fetus on karyotype analysis?

A. Neural tube defect
B. Fetal alcohol syndrome
C. Down syndrome
D. Edward syndrome
E. Patau syndrome

ANSWERS: What Would Gunner Jess/Jim Do?

1. WWGJD? A 16-year-old girl comes into the doctor's office for concern of amenorrhea. Her parents are worried that she has not yet had her period, even though her two sisters had menstrual cycles at the age of 13. The patient is self-conscious because her friends make fun of her for not having had any breast development. She thinks this is why she has never had a boyfriend. When the parents step out of the room, the girl states that she has never been sexually active and does not take any medications. On exam, she is fifth percentile for her age in height and has Tanner stage 1 breast development. There is a 2/6 holosystolic murmur that can be heard in the midsternal border. Her physical exam is otherwise normal. A urine pregnancy test is negative. What is the next best step in diagnosis?

Answer: C. Follicle-stimulating hormone level

Explanation: The patient's amenorrhea is most likely caused by streak ovaries from Turner syndrome (XO), as evidenced by her lack of secondary sexual characteristics (e.g., Tanner stage 1 breast development) and patent ductus arteriosus (e.g., {2/6} holosystolic murmur of the midsternal border). Once pregnancy is ruled out, the first step in the workup is an FSH level. If the FSH level is high (e.g., no estrogen being produced to inhibit it), it would be suggestive of Turner syndrome.

A. Transvaginal ultrasound (TVUS) → Incorrect. TVUS is not used to diagnose Turner syndrome.

B. Transabdominal ultrasound → Incorrect. Transabdominal ultrasound is not used to diagnose Turner syndrome, although it may be used to look for kidney defects.

D. Complete blood count (CBC) → Incorrect. Although a common laboratory test, a CBC would have no utility in the workup of Turner syndrome.

E. Karyotype analysis → Incorrect. Karyotype analysis is invasive and would only be considered once lab tests suggest the diagnosis of Turner syndrome (e.g., increased FSH levels) are performed.

2. WWGJD? A 16-year-old girl comes into the doctor's office because of her parent's concern of amenorrhea. Her mother had her period when she was 12 years-old and is concerned that her daughter is not developing as quickly. The patient is less concerned and states that she feels great. Unlike her friends, she never has to shave or use tampons. Her breast development is Tanner stage 3. Her physical exam reveals a short vaginal pouch with no palpable uterus or adnexa. Karyotype analysis shows 46XY. What is the most likely mechanism for her amenorrhea?

Answer: D. Defect of an androgen receptor

Explanation: The cause of this patient's amenorrhea is most likely AIS, which is caused by the defect of an androgen receptor. Patients with AIS have a 46XY genotype with a "short vaginal pouch" and no uterus, fallopian tube, or ovaries. In addition, they are hairless (e.g., "never has to shave"), but have normal breast development because free-floating androgens are converted into estrogen.

The easiest way to answer this question is to rule out based on genotype. Congenital adrenal hyperplasia (e.g., answer choices A and B) will present as 46XX. From there, you can differentiate based on the presence of hair. The only 46XY genotype disorder in which the patient is hairless is AIS.

A. Deficiency of 17-alpha hydroxylase → Incorrect. Patients with 17-alpha hydroxylase have delay in puberty that could lead to amenorrhea by the age of 16. However, the genotype is 46XX.

B. Defect in the *SRY* gene → Incorrect. Although patients may have a 46XY genotype, they can have hair growth because their androgen receptors are working. These patients require immediate removal of their gonads to PPx cancer. AIS patients only need removal of gonads after puberty.

C. 5-alpha reductase deficiency → Incorrect. Although patients with 5-alpha reductase deficiency have a 46XY genotype, the ambiguity of genitalia begins to change at the age of puberty. Thus, this patient would be expected to have development of more male sex characteristics, because testosterone can compensate for the lack of DHT.

E. Deficiency of 21-alpha hydroxylase → Incorrect. Patients with 21-alpha hydroxylase deficiency (CAH) have 46XX genotype if female external genitalia is present.

3. WWGJD? A 34-year-old, gravida 3, para 2, woman who is 17 weeks pregnant comes to the physician for a prenatal visit. During her visit she states that the swelling in her hands and feet are unchanged from the last time she was

seen. She gets very tired at times during the day but is still able to compelte her tasks at work. Last weekend, she accidentally had one sip of wine, but has not had any alcohol since the beginning of her pregnancy. The only medication she takes right now are folate supplements. She is still sexually active with her husband. Her vitals are 120/80 mm Hg, 90 bpm, 98.6°F, 14 RR. Her uterus is enlarged. Fetal heart rate is within normal limits. Her Quad screen results are:

Alpha fetoprotein: Decreased

Inhibin A: Increased

hCG: Increased

Estriol: Decreased

What is the most likely diagnosis of the fetus on karyotype analysis?

Answer: C. Down syndrome

Explanation: The Quad screen results suggest Down syndrome because the AFP and estriol are decreased and inhibin A and hCG are increased. Only three disorders are screened for on the Quad screen: neural tube defects (AFP increased), trisomy 21, and trisomy 18 (all decreased except for normal inhibin A). Patients carrying a fetus with Down syndrome should be counseled about future management.

A. Neural tube defect (NTD) → Incorrect. NTD would be expected if the AFP is increased.

B. Fetal alcohol syndrome → Incorrect. Fetal alcohol syndrome cannot be detected on Quad screen, and is usually only determined clinically.

D. Edward syndrome → Incorrect. The Quad screen would point to trisomy 18 if AFP, beta-hCG, and estriol were all decreased and inhibin A were normal. Newborns would be expected to have rocker-bottom feet, VSD, and overlapping fingers.

E. Patau syndrome → Incorrect. Trisomy 13 cannot be detected on the Quad screen. Newborns with Patau syndrome have polydactyly and cleft lip.

Adverse Effects of Drugs on Pregnancy, Childbirth, and the Puerperium

18

Kumar Nadhan, Hao-Hua Wu, and Leo Wang

Introduction

Teratogens are substances, often relatively innocuous to adults, with toxic effects on fetal development. When a mother is exposed to these substances during pregnancy, congenital abnormalities may develop, including physical malformation, mental or functional retardation, and death. The type and severity depends on the type and timing of the teratogen ingested. The parts of the human body forming embryologically at the time of ingestion are the most susceptible to insult. The obvious ideal management is primary prevention, best done by identifying risk factors for exposure. The test will challenge you in this manner, and provide you with clues as to which teratogen is most likely involved. When in doubt, it is always a safe bet to counsel a mother to discontinue a known teratogen.

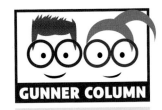

GUNNER COLUMN

Alcohol, Tobacco, and Other Drugs (ATODs)

Alcohol, tobacco, and other drugs (ATODs) mostly refers to commonly used, sometimes legal, drugs like alcohol and tobacco. There are many drugs in this category, but all of them follow the rule: Drugs are bad for the fetus. Help the mother stop doing drugs. Alcohol and tobacco use are most often seen in mothers who have a history of heavy use. Some mothers who did not plan on the pregnancy or have doubts about keeping the child may indulge in ATODs. Their feelings toward the baby must be addressed in prenatal visits. All mothers should be strictly counseled against ATOD use, but physicians may need to compromise, such as by minimizing instead of eliminating the number of cigarettes smoked daily.

Alcohol

Buzz Words: Short stature + normal karyotype + small face + thin upper lip/vermilion + no philtrum + mental retardation

Clinical Presentation: Alcohol during pregnancy leads to fetal alcohol syndrome (FAS), the leading cause of congenital mental retardation. FAS babies resemble Down syndrome babies; however, with the development of new

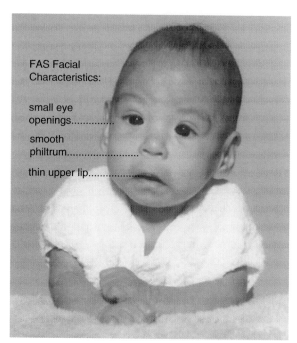

FIG. 18.1 Fetal alcohol syndrome (FAS) common identifiable features. (https://en.wikipedia.org/wiki/Fetal_alcohol_spectrum_disorder#/media/File:Photo_of_baby_with_FAS.jpg.)

technology, trisomy 21 is most likely found in utero. So if a child has a normal chromosomal screening but presents with Down syndrome–like features, that is a good hint!

Prophylaxis (PPx): Accurately assess and address the mother's alcohol consumption

Mechanism of Disease (MoD): Unknown

Diagnostic Steps (Dx):

1. Clinical, easiest to identify at birth.
2. Babies may show any combination of facial abnormalities: small skull size, small palpebral fishers, absent philtrum, thin upper and lower lips, and microcephaly.
3. What is less visible but may be present are organ development abnormalities: heart septal defects, malformed limbs, hearing impairment, gastrointestinal (GI), and renal defects (Fig. 18.1).

Treatment and Management Steps (Tx/Mgmt):

1. Early intervention for physical and mental defects
2. Supportive

Tobacco

Buzz Words: No hard drugs + miscarriage + unplanned pregnancy + low birth weight + sudden infant death syndrome (SIDS)

Clinical Presentation: A mother with a history of heavy tobacco use may present with premature rupture of membranes, placenta previa, placenta abruption, low birth weight, SIDS, cardiac defects.

PPx: Cessation of tobacco usage

MoD:

- Impaired umbilical cord function → decreased fetal oxygenation
- Nicotine → impaired lung development
- Carcinogens in cigarette → chromosomal instability

Dx:

1. Clinical presentation

Tx/Management:

1. Supportive

Prenatal Radiation Exposure

Radiation from medical imaging techniques can be split into ionizing and nonionizing radiation. Nonionizing radiation is relatively safe and includes microwaves and ultrasound. Magnetic resonance imaging (MRI), despite its loud scary noises, is also relatively safe. Thus, MRI and ultrasound are the best imaging modes for pregnant women. Ionizing radiation is more intense and teratogenic. This includes x-rays and, to a lesser extent, computed tomography (CT) scans. These modalities are still safe for fetuses but are preferably avoided. Patients may also receive radiation as therapy for cancer or thyroid disease, but this is usually stopped upon discovering the patient is pregnant. Rarely, radiation exposure may be from the environment, like working near an energy plant.

Buzz Words: Recent Emergency Department (ED) visit + hyperthyroidism + cancer + energy plant worker + imaging technician

Clinical Presentation: A first trimester (weeks 3–8) fetus is at highest risk from radiation damage and may present with mental and physical retardation. The parents may have a history of thyroid disease or multiple cancers in the family/nearby geographical area.

PPx: Avoid medical imaging

MoD: Radiation causes direct DNA structure damage and free radical formation.

Dx:

1. Clinical history and presentation

Tx/Management:

1. Avoid radiation during pregnancy.
2. Early intervention for physical and mental defects PTU for hyperthyroidism

TABLE 18.1 Major Teratogens

Teratogen	Affected Anatomy in Child	Risk Factor in Mother
ACE inhibitors/ARBs	Renal	HTN
Alkylating agents	Fingers	Chemotherapy
Aminoglycosides	Hearing	Pseudomonas
Anticonvulsants	Cleft lip/palate	Seizures
Cocaine	Placenta abruption, addiction	Addiction
DES	Vaginal clear cell adenocarcinoma	Breast cancer
Folate antagonists	CNS	Rheumatoid arthritis, cancer
Iodide	Cretinism	Hyperthyroidism
Lithium	Heart (Ebstein's anomaly)	Bipolar disorder
Maternal diabetes	Caudal regression syndrome, renal	Uncontrolled DM
Methimazole	Missing skin (aplasia cutis)	Hyperthyroidism
Phenytoin	Heart, cleft lip/palate	Seizures
Tetracyclines	Teeth	Bacterial infection, Lyme disease
Thalidomide	Limbs	Multiple myeloma, leprosy
Valproate	CNS	Seizures, bipolar disorder
Vitamin A	Abortion, multiple: eyes, heart, lungs	Acne treatment without OCP use
Warfarin	Abortion, hemorrhage, bones	DVT, PE, A-fib, valve, stroke

ACE, Angiotensin-converting enzyme; *A-fib,* atrial fibrillation; *ARBs,* angiotensin II receptor blockers; *CNS,* central nervous system; *DES,* diethylstilbestrol; *DM,* diabetes mellitus; *DVT,* deep vein thrombosis; *HTN,* hypertension; *PE,* pulmonary embolism.

Teratology (e.g., Angiotensin-Converting Enzyme [ACE] Inhibitors, Selective Serotonin Reuptake Inhibitors [SSRIs], Warfarin, Infections, Toxins)

Teratogen effects are varied based on the substance and timing of ingestion. A general rule is that teratogens taken during the first 3 weeks of gestation have the highest chance of leading to abortion. Weeks 3–8 host organogenesis, thus teratogens during this time will most likely result in one more organ malformations. Beyond week 8, expect to see growth and mental delay. Table 18.1 lists commonly tested teratogens. The most common effect of the teratogen (on the baby) is listed along with the risk factors or reasons why the mother would be exposed to the substance. Keep in mind, these are only the most commonly tested presentations.

GUNNER PRACTICE

1. A 23-year-old woman comes into your office worried because she thinks she has missed her period. It has been 5 weeks since her last menstrual period. The patient states that her cycle is strictly 4 weeks, with

occasional heavy bleeding. A pregnancy test is positive. She has a 4-year-old son, who is smaller than the other boys in his preschool. The patient is a current one-pack-per-day smoker and a social drinker. What is the most likely outcome for her current pregnancy?

A. Normal gestation and childbirth
B. Spontaneous abortion
C. Functional organ defect
D. Mental retardation
E. Twins

2. A 30-year-old woman with a history of breast cancer wants to have her first child. She has a history of breast cancer status post partial mastectomy, hypertension, and hyperthyroidism. She takes thiazide diuretics for her blood pressure and methimazole for her thyroid. What changes to her medications should you suggest she make?

A. No medication change
B. Switch thiazide to an ACE inhibitor
C. Switch thiazide to an angiotensin II receptor blocker (ARB)
D. Switch methimazole to PTU
E. Switch methimazole to potassium iodide

ANSWERS: What Would Gunner Jess/Jim Do?

1. WWGJD? A 23-year-old woman comes into your office worried because she thinks she has missed her period. It has been 5 weeks since her last menstrual period. The patient states her cycle is strictly 4 weeks, with occasional heavy bleeding. A pregnancy test is positive. She has a 4-year-old son, who is smaller than the other boys in his preschool. The patient is a current one-pack-per-day smoker and a social drinker. What is the most likely outcome for her current pregnancy?

Answer: A. Normal gestation and childbirth

Explanation: Although the patient ingests alcohol and smokes cigarettes, the most likely outcome is a normal course of pregnancy. Social drinking does not lead to FAS in the vast majority of patients, but the patient should be counseled to cease alcohol consumption. She should also be strictly counseled on smoking cessation, which would decrease the risk of spontaneous abortion. Spontaneous abortion outcomes befall a relatively high proportion but still a minority of smoking mothers. Low birth weight is a strong possibility for a pregnant mother who continues to smoke.

B. Spontaneous abortion → Incorrect. Spontaneous abortion is a worrisome risk of smoking in pregnant mothers, but is not the most likely outcome. This patient should be counseled on smoking cessation.

C. Functional organ defect → Incorrect. This is not the most likely outcome for light alcohol consumers, because they will most likely quit alcohol consumption during pregnancy with proper counseling. This is much more common if heavy alcohol consumption continues throughout the pregnancy. Smoking may lead to a low birth weight.

D. Mental retardation → Incorrect. Similar to functional organ defects, this is not the most likely outcome for light alcohol consumers, because they will most likely quit alcohol consumption during pregnancy with proper counseling. This is much more common if heavy alcohol consumption continues throughout the pregnancy.

E. Twins → Incorrect. Twinning is not associated with smoking or alcohol consumption.

2. WWGJD? A 30-year-old woman with a history of breast cancer wants to have her first child. She has a history of breast cancer status post partial mastectomy,

hypertension, and hyperthyroidism. She takes thiazide diuretics for her blood pressure and methimazole for her thyroid. What changes to her medications should you suggest she make?

Answer: D. Switch methimazole to PTU

Explanation: Methimazole is a hyperthyroid medication that is a teratogen. It most commonly leads to aplasia cutis, epidermal deficits, most commonly on the back of the head. PTU is a safe alternative used during pregnancy.

A. No medication change → Incorrect. Methimazole is a teratogen that must be discontinued.

B. Switch thiazide to ACE inhibitor → Incorrect. ACE inhibitors are teratogenic. Thiazide diuretics have been shown to be one of the least harmful antihypertensive therapies during pregnancy.

C. Switch thiazide to ARB → Incorrect. Like ACE inhibitors, ARBs are teratogenic. Both classes most commonly lead to renal abnormalities. They should not be used during pregnancy.

E. Switch methimazole to potassium iodide → Incorrect. Although methimazole should be discontinued, potassium iodide is not a safe alternative. Potassium iodide most commonly poses the risk of cretinism. Refer to Table 18.1 for further review.

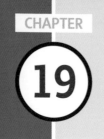

19

Systemic Disorders Affecting Pregnancy, Labor and Delivery, and the Puerperium

Gerald Michael Baer, Sierra Centokowski, Hao-Hua Wu, and Leo Wang

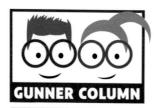

GUNNER COLUMN

Introduction

This chapter covers the high-yield medicine topics that will appear on your Ob/Gyn shelf. The key to answering these questions correctly on exam day is to know how the disease is relevant to pregnant patients. The most important organizing theme is that most of these disorders will have different treatment algorithms in a pregnant patient: Myasthenia gravis (MG) patients, for instance, cannot receive magnesium for the treatment of eclampsia; pregnant patients with hyperthyroidism need to be treated with propylthiouracil (PTU) instead of radioactive iodine. If you have taken other shelf exams before Ob/Gyn, feel free to peruse only the sections of the disease that pertain to pregnancy. Otherwise, become familiar with these buzz words and the order of diagnosis and management. The diseases covered in this chapter are all high-yield topics that are also seen on many other shelf exams.

Systemic Lupus Erythematosus (Lupus)

Buzz Words:

- RPR- and VDRL-positive + elevated PTT + recurrent abortions + malar rash → antiphospholipid antibody s/o systemic lupus erythematosus (SLE)
- Antihistone antibody + malar rash + new drug/medication → drug-induced lupus
- IgG + malar rash + discoid rash + antinuclear antibody (ANA) + mucositis (mouth ulcers) + neurologic dysfunction + serositis (pleuritis/pericarditis) + hematologic d/o (pancytopenia) + arthritis + renal d/o (wire loops) + photosensitivity + psychosis → SLE

Clinical Presentation: SLE is an autoimmune disorder that can present as nearly any chief complaint and is thus often kept somewhere on the differential. Importantly for the Ob/Gyn shelf, it can be associated with antiphospholipid antibodies, which can lead to recurrent spontaneous abortions. The classic presentation for SLE is a female

QUICK TIPS

Antiphospholipid antibodies include (1) lupus anticoagulant (elevates PTT), (2) anticardiolipin (fasle-positive VDRL and RPR), (3) anti-beta2-glycoprotein

QUICK TIPS

Antiphospholipid d/o characterized by hypercoagulable state due to antiphospholipid antibodies. Presents with recurrent pregnancy loss, stroke, and venous thrombosis. Treat with anticoagulation. Can be primary d/o or associated with SLE.

QUICK TIPS

Agents (e.g., slow acetylators in the liver) that lead to drug-induced lupus: SLE caused by sulfa HIPP-Es (Sulfa drugs, Hydralazine, Isoniazid, Procainamide, Phenytoin, Etanercept)

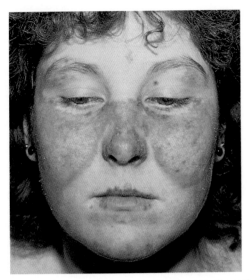

FIG. 19.1 Malar rash. (Lupus image bank, Elsevier: http://www.lupusimages.com/browser/detail/129/mucocutaneous-sle-malar-rash.)

patient with a malar (e.g., "butterfly") rash over the bridge of her nose who presents with constitutional symptoms, such as fatigue, fever, and night sweats (Fig. 19.1).

On the shelf, these patients typically have recently been exposed to sun (e.g., beach trip) or forgot to put on sunscreen. In addition, the shelf may try to trick you by showing either (1) lab results that falsely suggest syphilis (e.g., VDRL- and RPR-positive) or (2) lab results that falsely suggest a hematologic disorder (e.g., elevated PTT). Be very suspicious that these findings are due to antiphospholipid antibodies (e.g., lupus anticoagulant, etc.). For the Ob/Gyn shelf, these findings may present as a woman with a history of recurrent spontaneous abortions, a sequela of having circulating lupus anticoagulant. In addition, whenever someone is positive for anti-dsDNA or anti-Sm antibodies, know that is pathognomonic for SLE. SLE patients are also ANA-positive, but ANA is not specific for the disease. Finally, patients with antihistone antibodies have drug-induced lupus. Knowing these buzz words will help you avoid confusion and immediately sniff out what the National Board of Medical Examiners is up to.

Prophylaxis (PPx): Avoid sun exposure

Mechanism of Disease (MoD): Mostly considered a type 3 hypersensitivity because damage is mediated by antigen-antibody immune complexes.

- Sun damage → apoptotic debris → activation and production of antibodies that target antigens from

Lupus presentation video

the patient's cell nuclei → immune complex formed → immune complex deposited in body tissues → upregulates immune responses (using up complement proteins leading to deficient C1, C2, and C4)

- In pregnancy, **lupus anticoagulant** leads to thrombus development within the placenta → spontaneous abortion/pregnancy loss
- Pancytopenia in SLE is mediated by direct antibody attack on RBCs, WBCs, and platelets (type 2 hypersensitivity)

Diagnostic Steps (Dx):
1. ANA
2. Anti-Smith and anti-dsDNA antibodies (specific/gold standard for diagnosis)
3. Serum complement levels (may show decreased C1, C3, C4)

Treatment and Management Steps (Tx/Mgmt):
1. Nonsteroidal anti-inflammatory drugs (NSAIDs)
2. Steroids
3. Anticoagulation (e.g., warfarin, heparin) for antiphospholipid antibody syndrome
4. Discontinue drug if drug-induced lupus
5. Disease-modifying anti-inflammatory drugs (DMARDs) (e.g., methotrexate)
6. Biologics (e.g., tumor necrosis factor [TNF]-alpha inhibitors)
7. Renal transplant if kidney failure

Lupus treatment in pregnancy:
a. NSAIDs only for arthralgia/serositis and NOT for acute flares
b. Steroids for acute flares
c. Hydroxychloroquine → control skin manifestations; may cause lupus flare if d/c'd

Myasthenia Gravis

Buzz Words: Weakness of facial muscles + diplopia + worse with repeated activity, better with rest + ptosis with sustained upgaze + thymoma + acetylcholine receptor antibodies

Clinical Presentation: MG can be tested on the Ob/Gyn shelf because treatment may need to be altered during pregnancy. For instance, high-dose cyclosporine and azathioprine have been associated with low birth weight, preterm labor, and spontaneous abortion. Most importantly, giving **magnesium sulfate** to myasthenia patients with preeclampsia/eclampsia **is contraindicated** because it can precipitate a myasthenic crisis.

The predominant feature of MG is fluctuating weakness of the skeletal muscles, notably those of the face, throat, and neck. The key clinical features are weakness with repeated activity, gain in strength with rest, and improved strength with anticholinesterase drugs. Some MG patients will also have a thymic tumor.

PPx: Avoid **magnesium sulfate** for treatment of preeclampsia/eclampsia in pregnant patients with concomitant MG; instead, use valproic acid.

MoD:

- Autoantibodies generated to the acetylcholine receptor (on the postsynaptic side of the neuromuscular junction [NMJ]) → binding of autoantibodies blocks action of acetylcholine → antibody bindings leads to degradation of acetylcholine receptors → decreased binding sites + decreased number of receptors = lower amplitude of postsynaptic potentials at NMJ
- With repeated use, the amount of acetylcholine within the synaptic cleft decreases (less acetylcholine is released with each impulse), leading to weakness

Dx:

1. P/E showing weakness of facial muscles after sustained activity (ptosis with sustained upgaze).
2. Regained strength after period of rest.
3. Increased strength with acetylcholinesterase inhibitors (neostigmine and edrophonium).
4. Positive serum antiacetylcholine receptor antibodies (80%–90%).
5. Electromyography (EMG) showing reduced amplitude of muscle action potentials with repetitive stimulation.
6. Computed tomography (CT) of chest to evaluate for thymoma.

Tx/Mgmt:

1. Acetylcholinesterase inhibitors (neostigmine and pyridostigmine)
2. Immune-modulating agents like corticosteroids, azathioprine, cyclosporine (avoid high doses in pregnancy)
3. Plasma exchange (severe myasthenia refractory to acetylcholinesterase inhibitors/steroids)
4. Intravenous immunoglobulin (IVIG) (short-term control of worsening myasthenia)
5. Thymectomy (30% remission rate; perform in all patients with thymoma).
   - After delivery, **infants should be monitored** for signs of MG, as there may be transient symptoms.
   - For myasthenic crisis, secure airway, ventilate, and initiate plasma exchange/IVIG. Start

QUICK TIPS

Acetylcholinesterase inhibitors mechanism of action (MoA) = decrease destruction of acetylcholine in synaptic left; more acetylcholine = stronger postsynaptic amplitude and better contraction anticholinesterase inhibitors and steroids as the patient is weaning from ventilator.

Hyperthyroidism

Buzz Words: Heat intolerance (excessive sweating or "hot flashes") + insomnia + anxiety + weight loss, arrhythmias + proptosis + middle-aged female + pretibial myxedema

Clinical Presentation: Thyroid disorders are often tested on the Ob/Gyn shelf because thyroid labs can be abnormal in normal pregnancy. Thus it is important to differentiate normal from abnormal. In normal pregnancy, **total** T4 andT3 are elevated. However, there is no change in **free** T4, T3, and thyroid-stimulating hormone (TSH). In contrast, in hyperthyroidism, TSH is decreased secondary to inhibition from high levels of **free T4.** In addition, it is also important to note the differences in treatment between nonpregnant and pregnant females. For nonpregnant females, hyperthyroidism can be treated with methimazole and radioactive iodine (I-131). For **pregnant patients, PTU is the treatment of choice.**

PPx: N/A

MoD:

- Hyperthyroidism can result from a number of causes, including Graves disease (autoimmune disorder), thyroiditis, and a hyperfunctioning nodule.
- Mechanism of proptosis and pretibial myxedema: TSH receptors in fibroblasts in the eye and lower leg → activation of TSH receptors → buildup of glycosaminoglycan in lower leg and eye.

Dx:

1. TSH with reflux to T4, radioactive iodine uptake
   - Low TSH, high T4, increased uptake of radioactive iodine (I-123).
   - If both TSH and T4 are increased, consider secondary hyperthyroidism caused by pituitary, which is very rare.
   - Note: Order pregnancy test for increased thyroid-binding globulin (TBG) and low radioactive T3 uptake.

Tx/Mgmt:

1. Beta blocker (propranolol) for immediate management of adrenergic symptoms.
2. Methimazole (thionamide; inhibits conversion of T4 to T3).
3. PTU for pregnant patients:
   - Avoid methimazole and I-131 in pregnant patients.

AR

Proptosis = bulging eyes

99 AR

Pretibial myxedema is swelling of the lower legs due to increased buildup of glycosaminoglycan

FOR THE WARDS

Graves disease is due to an autoantibody that stimulates the thyroid receptor for TSH → excess T4 and T3.

Hypothyroidism

Buzz Words: Cold intolerance + fatigue + weakness + brady-cardia + goiter + dry skin

Clinical Presentation: Less commonly tested than hyperthy-roidism on the Ob/Gyn shelf but good to know to rule out answer choices. Hypothyroidism is a disorder of decreased free T3 and T4, leading to cold intolerance, fatigue, weakness, and bradycardia.

PPx: N/A

MoD: Can be due to chronic autoimmune hypothyroidism (Hashimoto), whereby thyroid peroxidase (TPO) anti-bodies destroy thyroid, or to iodine insufficiency.

Dx:
1. TSH with reflux to T4 (shows high TSH, low T4)
2. Enzyme-linked immunosorbent assay (ELISA) to look for antibodies (e.g., antimicrosomal antibodies or TPO antibodies)

Tx/Mgmt:
1. Levothyroxine

Appendicitis

Buzz Words: Young adult female + umbilical pain that migrates to right lower quadrant (RLQ) + acute + leukocytosis + peritoneal signs + fever + **refuses to eat** + negative urine pregnancy test → appendicitis

Clinical Presentation: On the OB/Gyn shelf, young female adult patients with acute RLQ pain can either have appendici-tis or ectopic pregnancy. To differentiate, a urine preg-nancy test is ordered (positive = ectopic pregnancy). Appendicitis patients can present with nausea and vomiting (N/V), aversion to food, and dull epigastric pain that migrates to McBurney's point; can also have posi-tive Rovsing sign (palpation of left lower quadrant [LLQ] increases pain at RLQ), psoas sign (pain with extension of iliopsoas muscle, aka hip extension), and obturator sign (pain with flexion and internal rotation of the hip).

PPx: N/A

MoD: Obstruction of the lumen of the appendix is the most common cause of inflammation. Fecaliths, undigested seeds, pinworm infections, or lymphoid hyperplasia may be the cause of obstruction. Once occluded, the epithelial lining continues to secrete mucus until the intraluminal pressure occludes venous outflow. Venous congestion and intraluminal stasis set the stage for bac-terial overgrowth and progressive inflammation.

Dx:
1. Pulmonary embolism (PE)
2. If reproductive-age female, beta-hCG to r/o ectopic pregnancy
3. CT to confirm acute appendicitis
4. If pregnant or a pediatric patient, U/S or MRI preferred

Tx/Mgmt:
1. Appendectomy
2. Antibiotics
3. If cancer at base of appendix → right hemicolectomy

Carpal Tunnel Syndrome

Buzz Words: Pregnant + hyper/hypothyroid + repetitive hand work + pain in wrist/hand at night + numbness/tingling of fingers + positive Phalen or Tinel sign + thenar atrophy

Clinical Presentation: Carpal tunnel syndrome (CTS) is a commonly tested disorder on the Ob/Gyn shelf because it integrates knowledge from multiple different specialties (e.g., Medicine, Surgery, and Neurology). During pregnancy, patients can experience new CTS or exacerbation of chronic CTS due to distal swelling of the upper extremity. For the shelf, know the sequence of diagnostic and treatment steps (e.g., patient has already tried rest, splint, and NSAIDs. What is the next best treatment?), as this is likely to be at least one question on exam day.

PPx: Avoid repetitive wrist motion (e.g., extensive flexion and extension)

MoD: Swelling of soft tissues due to edema from pregnancy → compression of the median nerve in the carpal tunnel of the wrist. In addition to pregnancy, CTS is also associated with hypo/hyperthyroidism, acromegaly, diabetes, and dialysis-related amyloidosis.

Dx:
1. Clinical exam.
2. Wrist XR to r/o fractures/arthritis (make sure to use lead to protect fetus from radiation).
3. **Nerve conduction studies** are the most likely to confirm the diagnosis.
4. Electromyography (if surgery is required).
5. MRI only if EMG is equivocal (CT not needed until after delivery of baby).

Tx/Mgmt:
1. Rest

99 AR

Phalen and Tinel's signs

99 AR

Carpal tunnel syndrome

2. Wrist splint
3. Acetaminophen for pain (avoid NSAIDs as they can close ductus arteriosus)
4. Corticosteroid shots (effective in 80%–90% of patients but may return after months; should not be given >3 times a year)
5. Surgery (carpal tunnel release) as last resort (must have EMG beforehand)

Pubic Symphysis Separation

Buzz Words: Pregnant patient + suprapubic pain and tenderness + swelling/edema of the pubic symphysis

Clinical Presentation: In normal pregnancy, the pubic symphysis and the sacroiliac joints widen to prepare for delivery of the fetus. However, the widening may become pathologic when the patient experiences pain and swelling exacerbated by weight bearing, making activities of daily living difficult. The diagnosis can be made clinically (e.g., suprapubic tenderness and swelling on PE). An XR showing a widening of 10–13 mm on imaging can be used to make the diagnosis but is not necessary and should be avoided to prevent fetal radiation exposure.

PPx: N/A

MoD: Ligamentous laxity at pubic symphysis during pregnancy → separation at pubic symphysis

Dx:
1. Clinical presentation
2. Pelvic XR (but not needed for the diagnosis!)

Tx/Mgmt:
1. Acetaminophen for pain (no NSAIDs for fear of closing the ductus areteriosus)
2. Pelvic brace
3. Cane or crutch to support ambulation
4. Physical therapy

Venous Thromboembolism (VTE) in Pregnancy

Buzz Words:
- Postpartum s/p C-section + pleuritic chest pain + shortness of breath + tachycardia + hypoxia → PE
- During pregnancy or postpartum s/p C-section + calf swelling + collateral superficial veins present + pain with dorsiflexion of ankle (Homans sign) + pitting edema → deep venous thrombosis (DVT)

99 AR

Pubic symphysis separation images

QUICK TIPS

Remember Wells' criteria for DVT

Clinical Presentation: VTE is high-yield because it is one of the leading causes of maternal mortality during or after pregnancy. Pregnancy is a hypercoagulable state because of stasis in lower extremities, which increases the risk of DVTs and PEs. For DVTs, the patient can present either during pregnancy (e.g., period of immobility) or after C-section (s/p surgery) with unilateral calf pain exacerbated by ankle dorsiflexion. There may also be increased swelling compared with the contralateral side. Diagnosis of DVT is confirmed with Doppler ultrasound.

On the shelf, patients with a PE will present within a week after a C-section with shortness of breath, pleuritic chest pain, and hypoxia. If it is a saddle, the patient could become **hemodynamically unstable.**

PPx: Avoid long periods of immobility as well as surgical management. Use compression boots.

MoD: Stasis of blood in lower extremity → hypercoagulability → clot formation

Dx:

1. For DVT: Physical exam + Doppler ultrasound of venous system of affected limb
2. For PE: Physical exam + D-dimer + CT angiography

Tx/Mgmt:

1. Oxygen therapy
2. Enoxaparin
3. Heparin (avoid warfarin in pregnant patients, since it can cause skeletal abnormalities and a hypoplastic nose)

GUNNER PRACTICE

1. A 35-year-old, gravida 3, para 3, woman is found to be short of breath and with chest pain at 33 weeks' gestation. She states that the chest pain is sharp and increases with inhalation. Her vitals are 100/60 mm Hg, 110 bpm, 99°F, 24 RR, and 89% on room air. Wheezing can be heard on auscultation. She is placed on 6 L of O_2. Arterial blood gas shows a pH of 7.30 and a pCO_2 of 30 mm Hg. What is the most appropriate treatment for this patient's symptoms?
   A. Albuterol
   B. Heparin
   C. Warfarin
   D. Enoxaparin
   E. Expectant management

2. A 31-year-old, gravida 2, para 1, woman at 19 weeks' gestation presents to her doctor with right wrist pain. She states the pain in her wrist gets worse during the day when she is typing up documents at work and sometimes wakes her up in the middle of the night. The pain is also sometimes associated with numbness that shoots up to her thumb. She has tried rest and acetaminophen without any benefit. On exam, pain and paresthesia are reproduced when the center of her wrist is tapped. What is the next best step in the management of this condition?
   A. Ibuprofen
   B. Naproxen
   C. Wrist splint
   D. Corticosteroid injection
   E. Carpal tunnel release

3. A 30-year-old, gravida 2, para 1, woman at 30 weeks' gestation visits her doctor, reporting increasing agitation and diaphoresis over the previous week. She states that she can feel her heart racing out of her chest, and this only increases her anxiety. Although she has a history of having used cocaine in her early 20s, she denies using any drugs during the course of her pregnancy. Now she takes only folate supplements. Her vitals are 150/100 mm Hg, 120 bpm, 99°F, 24 RR, and 97% on room air. On exam, she has an enlarged, nontender thyroid, and swelling of her lower legs as well as bulging of her right eyeball. Complete blood count is normal. Beta-blockers are administered to control blood pressure. Thyroid labs are sent. What is the next best step in managing this patient's symptoms?
   A. Radioactive iodine
   B. Potassium iodine
   C. Methimazole
   D. Propylthiouracil therapy
   E. Lorazepam

ANSWERS: What Would Gunner Jess/Jim Do?

1. WWGJD? A 35-year-old, gravida 3, para 2, woman is found to be short of breath and chest pain at 33 weeks' gestation. She states that the chest pain is sharp and increases with inhalation. Her vitals are 100/60 mm Hg, 110 bpm, 99°F, 24 RR, and 89% on room air. Wheezing can be heard on auscultation. She is placed on 6 L of O_2. Arterial blood gas shows a pH of 7.30, a pCO_2 of 30 mm Hg. What is the most appropriate treatment for this patient's symptoms?

Answer: D. Enoxaparin

Explanation: The patient's symptoms of shortness of breath and pleuritic chest pain as well as her tachycardia and hypoxia are indicative of pulmonary embolism (PE). Pregnancy increases the risk for venous thromboembolism because it is a hypercoagulable state. After O_2 administration, enoxaparin is preferred for treatment because it does not cross the placental barrier.

A. Albuterol → Incorrect. Albuterol is a short-acting beta agonist and is used to treat asthma. It is also safe for use in pregnancy but is not a treatment for PE.

B. Heparin → Incorrect. Heparin can also be used to treat PE in pregnancy but is second-line to enoxaparin.

C. Warfarin → Incorrect. Warfarin should not be used owing to its teratogenicity. In patients who are not pregnant, warfarin is the preferred treatment.

E. Expectant management → Incorrect. PE is an emergent condition and should be treated accordingly.

2. WWGJD? A 31-year-old, gravida 2, para 1, woman at 19 weeks' gestation presents to her doctor with right wrist pain. She states the pain in her wrist gets worse during the day when she is typing up documents at work and sometimes wakes her up in the middle of the night. The pain is also sometimes associated with numbness that shoots up to her thumb. Patient has tried rest and acetaminophen without any benefit. On exam, pain and paresthesia is reproduced when the center of her wrist is tapped. What is the next best step in the management of this disease?

Answer: C. Wrist splint

Explanation: This patient has carpal tunnel syndrome (CTS), as evidenced by the wrist pain and shooting numbness in the distribution of the median nerve.

For pregnant patients, the first-line treatment for CTS is a wrist splint, which stabilizes the wrist and reduces compression of the carpal tunnel. Nonsteroidal anti-inflammatory drugs (NSAIDs) are not indicated in a pregnant patient because of the risk of closing the ductus arteriosus.

A. Ibuprofen → Incorrect. Avoid NSAIDs in pregnancy because of the risk of ductus arteriosus closure.

B. Naproxen → Incorrect. Avoid NSAIDs in pregnancy because of risk of ductus arteriosus closure.

D. Corticosteroid injection → Incorrect. This would be the next step in treatment after a wrist splint and acetaminophen.

E. Surgical carpal tunnel release → Incorrect. Elective surgical management should always be the treatment of last resort on the shelf.

3. **WWGJD?** A 30-year-old, gravida 2, para 1, woman at 30 weeks' gestation comes to her doctor with increasing agitation and diaphoresis over the past week. She states that she can feel her heart racing out of her chest, and this only increases her anxiety. Although she has a history of cocaine use in her early twenties, she denies using any drugs during the course of her pregnancy. The only thing she takes right now are folate supplements. Her vitals are 150/100 mm Hg, 120 bpm, 99°F, 24 RR, and 97% on room air. On exam, she has an enlarged, nontender thyroid, and swelling of her lower legs as well as bulging of her right eyeball. Complete blood count is normal. Beta-blockers are administered to control blood pressure. Thyroid labs are sent. What is the next best step in managing this patient's symptoms?

Answer: D. Propylthiouracil therapy

Explanation: For medical conditions tested on the Ob/Gyn shelf, be on the lookout for questions about treatment, since many times the preferred treatment for a disease can be contraindicated in a pregnant patient. In this question stem, the patient has hyperthyroidism, as shown by the buzz words "swelling of her lower legs" (pretibial myxedema) and "bulging of her right eyeball" (proptosis). Treatment involves beta-blockers first to control blood pressure and then propylthiouracil (PTU) therapy for maintenance. For nonpregnant patients, the answer would probably be radioactive iodine.

A. Radioactive iodine → Incorrect. Contraindicated during pregnancy, although the preferred treatment option for hyperthyroidism in a nonpregnant patient.

B. Potassium iodine → Incorrect. Used to replete iodide in **hypo**thyroidism.

C. Methimazole → Incorrect. Also not used in pregnancy due to side effects (agranulocytosis).

E. Lorazepam → Incorrect. Although the patient appears anxious, her anxiety is due to her underlying hyperthyroidism, which is not addressed by lorazepam.

Gunner Jim's Guide to Exam Day Success

Leo Wang and Hao-Hua Wu

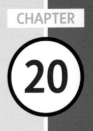

20

Do these three things to perform well on any shelf:
1. Master one review book.
2. Do as many quality questions as you can.
3. Review questions on Excel.

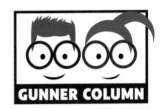

GUNNER COLUMN

"Master One Review Book"

The Ob/Gyn clerkship rotation ranges from 4 to 8 weeks (typically 6). That is not enough time to peruse multiple review books. The most important thing you can do prior to the start of your rotation is to identify the resource that best covers the material of the Pediatrics shelf, such as *Gunner Goggles Obstetrics and Gynecology*. Once you have picked something, stick with it. The point of using a review book is hat you can become familiar with the scope of the exam.

Most of your learning takes place when you complete questions, so don't be discouraged if you cannot memorize every word of your review book, as you did for step 1. Instead, use this review book as a point of reference and annotate the margins.

If you see one topic come up in multiple chapters (or maybe even multiple shelf exams), make sure to write down the page numbers where it appears and flip to those pages every time you review. The more connections you make between topics (e.g., thinking of syphilis as a disease process that can present as a dermatologic complaint [painless ulcer, palm/sole rash, gummas] and a neurologic complaint [neurosyphilis]), the more you will master.

In addition, highlight themes that keep coming up. For instance, anytime patients in the question recently change their medication regimen, suspect the medication change as the cause of their symptoms until proven otherwise. These organizing principles transcend individual topics and can help you do well on any shelf exam test question.

"Do as Many Quality Questions as You Can"

The key to success is practicing in an environment that simulates the pressure of test day. And nothing simulates that pressure better than taking practice questions under stringent time constraints.

After you identify your review book, select as many authoritative question banks as you can. We recommend Gunner Practice, UWorld, and National Board of Medical Examiners (NBME) Clinical Science practice exams. Do at least 10 questions a day under timed conditions (1.5 minutes a question) starting on the first day of your rotation.

Remember, you can complete the same question multiple times in the course of study! In fact, it is recommended that you retry the questions you got wrong in the first place, just so that you know you would get it right on the test.

It is also important that the questions you complete are of high quality. This means that the length and content of the question stems reflect what you would actually see on test day. Many question bank resources are too easy (giving you a false sense of confidence) or ask about material that would not show up on the exam (wasting your time).

Once you have selected your question bank resources, count the total number of questions and divide it by the number of days you have available to study. Then make sure you set a study plan where you can make at least two passes through your questions. The first pass is completion of all available questions. The second pass is completion of all the questions you got wrong or made a lucky guess on during your first pass. Seeing how many of the second-pass questions you get correct should be a nice confidence booster leading into exam day.

"Review Questions on Excel"

How you take notes for the questions you complete is imperative to success.

The most effective strategy is to pick **one** take-home point for every question you complete and record it on an Excel spreadsheet specific to your clinical rotation.

For instance, if you gave a wrong answer to a question about the treatment of bacterial vaginosis, write "Tx of bacterial vaginosis" in column A and then "metronidazole" in column B of your Excel spreadsheet. This will allow you to create an immediate "flashcard." When you review this material the following week, you can put your cursor over column A, say the answer out loud, and check your answer by shifting your cursor to column B. This will save you a lot of time and jump directly the most important take-away for each question.

If you understand everything in the question and answer choices, don't record it on the Excel spreadsheet.

If you don't understand multiple things in the question and answer choices, record the most important takeaway point and move on. For test day, it is better to be confident in what you know well than to undermine your confidence by fixating on what you are weak at.

By test day, you should have one Excel spreadsheet that contains one important take-home point for every question you were unsure about. The tabs on the bottom should be organized by question-bank resource. This Excel spreadsheet would ideally take only 3 to 4 hours to review, and it is something you would go over the day before the exam.

In Summary: Read, Apply, and Review

And prepare for success on test day!

Index

Note: 'Page numbers followed by "f" indicate figures, "t" indicate tables "b" indicate boxes.'